Washington MPJE® Exam Prep

200 Pharmacy Law Practice Questions

- ☑ 100 FEDERAL LAW QUESTIONS
- ☑ 100 WASHINGTON STATE LAW QUESTIONS

PHARMACY TESTING SOLUTIONS   2024 EDITION

ISBN: 979-8-8362-5549-7

Table of Contents

Introduction

The Multistate Pharmacy Jurisprudence Examination, or MPJE, is the pharmacy law exam created by the National Association of Boards of Pharmacy. It is designed to test your knowledge and competency of pharmacy law. The exam consists of 120 federal and state-specific questions that cover three content areas: pharmacy practice (83% of the questions); licensure, registration, certification, and operational requirements (15% of the questions); and general regulatory processes (2% of the questions).

This book will help you prepare for federal and state questions from all content areas. The first section includes 100 questions on federal pharmacy law. The second section includes 100 questions on Washington state pharmacy law. At the back of the book is an answer index with detailed explanations for each question. When taking the MPJE, it is important to choose the most strict answer if there are differences between federal and state laws (unless otherwise instructed to answer specifically federal or state law).

When preparing for the MPJE, remove all distractions, read each question carefully, and try not to refer to any resources. The actual exam is 2½ hours, so you might find it helpful to time yourself to ensure you are not taking too much (or too little) time on each question.

Make sure to spread out your study time as well; cramming the night before an exam is proven to result in low retention and difficulty focusing during the test. Study gradually over time and test your competency and timing using this book.

On the day of the exam, make sure you are well rested, you eat a substantial breakfast, and you leave for the testing center early, so that you will arrive at least 30 minutes before the exam starts. Good luck on the MPJE, and happy studying!

Federal MPJE Practice Questions

1. What was the first law requiring drugs to be proven safe before being marketed?
    a. Food, Drug, and Cosmetic Act
    b. Kefauver-Harris Amendment
    c. Pure Food and Drug Act
    d. Prescription Drug Marketing Act
    e. Durham-Humphrey Amendment

2. A pharmacist receives an urgent notification from a manufacturing company for a recall of a specific medication because it may cause serious adverse health issues or death. What type of drug recall is this?
    a. Class I
    b. Class II
    c. Class III
    d. Class IV
    e. Class V

3. What agency is responsible for the federal Controlled Substances Act (CSA)?
    a. Federal Bureau of Investigation (FBI)
    b. Food and Drug Administration (FDA)
    c. Department of Health and Human Services (HHS)
    d. Drug Enforcement Administration (DEA)
    e. United States Pharmacopeia (USP)

4. A pharmacist wants to know if generic warfarin tablets are bioequivalent to brand name Coumadin tablets. Where can this information be found?
   a. The Purple Book
   b. The Blue Book
   c. The Green Book
   d. The Orange Book
   e. The Red Book

5. Which of the following is NOT required on the manufacturer's drug container label for an oral drug product?
   a. Name of the manufacturer
   b. Expiration date
   c. Name of the drug or product
   d. Directions for administration
   e. Net quantity packaged

6. According to federal law, what age must the purchaser be to purchase a controlled substance without a prescription that contains opium?
   a. 16
   b. 18
   c. 21
   d. 25
   e. No age requirement

7. Which DEA form must be completed and submitted to the DEA upon discovering a theft or significant loss of controlled substances?
   a. DEA Form 106
   b. DEA Form 108
   c. DEA Form 222
   d. DEA Form 224
   e. DEA Form 363

8. Which of the following is a Schedule II controlled substance?
   a. Buprenorphine
   b. Butabarbital
   c. Mescaline
   d. Pentobarbital
   e. Modafinil

9. A water-containing oral formulation that is compounded from commercially available drug products has a maximum beyond-use-date (BUD) of _____ when refrigerated.
    a. 3 days
    b. 7 days
    c. 14 days
    d. 30 days
    e. 45 days

10. Practitioners who dispense methadone for detoxification must register for a narcotic treatment program using what form?
    a. DEA Form 222
    b. DEA Form 224
    c. DEA Form 363
    d. DEA Form 106
    e. DEA Form 41

11. Which FDA expedited review program is intended for drugs that treat serious conditions and fill an unmet medical need?
    a. Breakthrough therapy
    b. Instant approval
    c. Fast track
    d. Accelerated approval
    e. Priority review

12. Schedule II controlled substances CANNOT be transferred in which of the following scenarios?
    a. A pharmacy is closing and decides to transfer their Schedule II controlled substance inventory to another pharmacy
    b. A pharmacy is not renewing their DEA registration and therefore wants to transfer their remaining Schedule II controlled substances to another pharmacy
    c. A pharmacy ordered the wrong Schedule II controlled substances and wants to transfer them back to the supplier
    d. A researcher would like to transfer excess Schedule II controlled substances to a pharmacy to be dispensed to patients
    e. A pharmacy wants to transfer 2 bottles of Schedule II controlled substances to another pharmacy

13. A patient wants to refill a prescription but was not satisfied with the pharmacy that filled and dispensed the prescription the first time. The patient demands the prescription be returned so they can take it to a different pharmacy to obtain refills. The pharmacist should:
    a. Document the original fill information on the original prescription, keep a copy, and return the original prescription to the patient
    b. Offer to give a copy of the prescription to the patient, keep the original copy at the pharmacy, and recommend the patient request the prescription be transferred to another pharmacy if legal
    c. Void the original prescription before returning it to the patient and offer to transfer the rest verbally to another pharmacy
    d. Document the situation in the patient's profile and return the original prescription to the patient
    e. Inform the patient you can send the prescription by priority mail to the pharmacy of their choice

14. When a pharmacy submits a DEA Form 222 (single sheet) to purchase Schedule II controlled substances, who keeps the original copy of the DEA Form 222?
    a. The pharmacy
    b. The supplier
    c. The manufacturer
    d. The DEA
    e. The pharmacist

15. For which type of drug recall is there a possibility of temporary or medically reversible adverse effects, but the probability of serious adverse effects is remote?
    a. Class I
    b. Class II
    c. Class III
    d. Class A
    e. Class B

16. A drug has an NDC of 16103-0350-11. The 0350 represents:
    a. The manufacturer name
    b. The amount packaged
    c. The identity of the drug
    d. The location of manufacturing
    e. The route of administration

17. What set of regulations specifies the required minimum manufacturing standards for pharmaceutical products in the U.S.?
    a. Standards of Manufacturing Practice (SMP)
    b. Good Pharmaceutical Manufacturing Practice (GPMP)
    c. Requirements of Good Manufacturing Practice (RGMP)
    d. Regulations of Manufacturing Practice (RMP)
    e. Good Manufacturing Practice (GMP)

18. A prescriber may issue multiple prescriptions authorizing a patient to receive a total of up to a 90-day supply of a Schedule II controlled substance if certain conditions are met. Which of the following is NOT one of those conditions?
    a. Each separate prescription must be issued for a legitimate medical purpose
    b. The prescriber must include written instructions on each consecutive prescription indicating the earliest month in which a pharmacy may fill it
    c. The prescriber must conclude that providing the patient with multiple prescriptions will not create an undue risk of diversion or abuse
    d. The issuance of multiple prescriptions must be permissible under the applicable state law
    e. The prescriber must comply fully with all other applicable requirements

19. A prescription for lorazepam can be refilled a maximum of how many times within a six-month period?
    a. Zero
    b. Two
    c. Three
    d. Five
    e. Six

20. In order for buprenorphine to be prescribed, which of the following conditions must be met?
    a. The prescriber's liability insurance must provide buprenorphine indemnity
    b. The prescriber must have less than 30 patients to whom they prescribe buprenorphine
    c. The prescriber must have been granted a waiver from the DEA in order to prescribe buprenorphine
    d. The prescriber must have an active DEA license that includes the schedule in which buprenorphine is listed
    e. The prescriber must have an active "X" number

21. An example of an adulterated drug is:
    a. The name of the manufacturer is not included on the label
    b. A medication that has an unapproved color additive
    c. Active ingredients are missing from the bottle
    d. The drug causes an allergic reaction in the patient
    e. The drug container does not contain proper directions for nonprescription drugs

22. Which of the following is a mid-level practitioner?
    a. Physician
    b. Dentist
    c. Veterinarian
    d. Optometrist
    e. Podiatrist

23. Durable Medical Equipment (DME) must meet which standard(s)? Select ALL that apply.
    a. Can withstand repeated use
    b. Strictly for assistance with walking
    c. Limited to use for paraplegics
    d. Appropriate for use in the home
    e. Primarily for a medical purpose

24. What act regulates the sale and recordkeeping requirements for prescription drug samples?
    a. Prescription Drug Marketing Act
    b. Durham-Humphrey Amendment
    c. Pure Food and Drug Act
    d. Food, Drug and Cosmetic Act
    e. Kefauver-Harris Amendment

25. Which of the following can be determined from the National Drug Code (NDC) number on a medication bottle? Select ALL that apply.
    a. Manufacturer
    b. Specific drug
    c. Package
    d. Expiration date
    e. FDA approval status

26. Under the iPLEDGE Risk Evaluation and Mitigation Strategy (REMS) for isotretinoin, what is the maximum number of refills that may be authorized on a prescription?
    a. 0 refills
    b. 1 refill
    c. 2 refills
    d. 5 refills
    e. 11 refills

27. In which situation would it be illegal for a pharmacy to compound drugs?
    a. The quantity prepared is reasonable for filling existing and anticipated prescriptions
    b. Dosage forms are sold only to other pharmacies and not physician offices
    c. Ingredients in the compounded drugs meet national standards
    d. The compounded drug is not commercially available
    e. Interstate distribution of compounded drugs is no more than 5% of total prescriptions sold by the pharmacy per year

28. What DEA form is necessary to purchase or transfer Schedule II controlled substances?
    a. DEA Form 108
    b. DEA Form 222
    c. DEA Form 224
    d. DEA Form 225
    e. DEA Form 363

29. A patient calls the pharmacy and says they just got home from the hospital after having broken their leg. The patient cannot make it to the pharmacy to pick up their prescription for a Schedule II controlled substance that is ready to pick up. The patient asks if the pharmacy can mail the prescription to the house (mail delivery). How should the pharmacist respond?
    a. Controlled substance medications cannot be mailed
    b. Only Schedule III–V controlled substances can be mailed
    c. Controlled substances can only be mailed to the prescriber's office for office pickup
    d. The prescription can be sent to the patient through the mail
    e. The prescription can be sent to the patient as long as the drug name is listed on the package

30. Which of the following statements is/are true about narrow therapeutic index (NTI) drugs?

    I.   Small differences in the dose or blood concentration may lead to adverse reactions

    II.   They are not permitted to be prescribed

    III.   They require careful titration or patient monitoring for safe and effective use

    a. I only
    b. II only
    c. I and III only
    d. II and III only
    e. I, II, and III

31. What act set the requirement for child-resistant closures for prescription drugs, non-prescription drugs, and hazardous household products?
    a. Poison Prevention Packaging Act
    b. Child Drug Safety Act
    c. Prevention of Hazardous Consumption Act
    d. Children Poison Prevention Act
    e. Hazardous Materials Safety Act

32. According to the Combat Methamphetamine Epidemic Act of 2005, the logbook requirement does NOT apply to individual single sales of packages of:
    a. No more than 60mg of pseudoephedrine
    b. No less than 60mg of pseudoephedrine
    c. No more than 50mg of pseudoephedrine
    d. No less than 50mg of pseudoephedrine
    e. All pseudoephedrine sales are required to be logged

33. Over-the-counter (OTC) drug advertising is regulated by the:
    a. Federal Trade Commission
    b. Food and Drug Administration
    c. Drug Quality and Security Commission
    d. Consumer Product Safety Commission
    e. None of the above

34. What information is required to be included in the transaction report transmitted from a manufacturer to a pharmacy when the pharmacy purchases bulk bottles of a medication?
    a. Transaction information, transaction history, transaction log
    b. Transaction purpose, transaction history, transaction ID number
    c. Transaction information, transaction history, transaction statement
    d. Transaction ID number, transaction code, transaction statement
    e. Transaction purpose, transaction history, transaction log

35. What law requires drugs to be proven effective (as well as safe) before being marketed?
    a. Durham-Humphrey Amendment
    b. Pure Food and Drug Act
    c. Prescription Drug Marketing Act
    d. Hatch-Waxman Amendment
    e. Kefauver-Harris Amendment

36. Which DEA registration form is used for pharmacies to register with the DEA to possess and dispense controlled substances?
    a. DEA Form 106
    b. DEA Form 222
    c. DEA Form 224
    d. DEA Form 225
    e. DEA Form 363

37. Re-importation of medications is only legal if performed by the:

    I. Retail pharmacy

    II. Original manufacturer

    III. Wholesale distributor

    a. I only
    b. II only
    c. III only
    d. I and III only
    e. I, II, and III

38. Which of the following is true regarding the stocking and dispensing of methadone at retail pharmacies?
    a. Methadone may not be stocked or dispensed from a retail pharmacy; patients must obtain methadone from a narcotic treatment facility
    b. Methadone may be stocked at a retail pharmacy, but may only be dispensed as an analgesic
    c. Methadone may be stocked at a retail pharmacy, but may only be dispensed for narcotic dependence
    d. Methadone may be stocked at a retail pharmacy and may be dispensed as either an analgesic or for the short-term treatment of narcotic dependence
    e. Methadone may be stocked at any pharmacy and may be dispensed as either an analgesic or for the long-term treatment of narcotic dependence

39. What act requires health care facilities to report death or injuries caused by or suspected to have been caused by a medical device to the FDA or the manufacturer?
    a. FDA Modernization Act
    b. Medical Device Inspection Act
    c. Safe Medical Device Act
    d. Pure Food and Drug Act
    e. The Omnibus Budget Reconciliation Act

40. An example of a misbranded manufacturer's container of a drug would be:
    a. The drug causes an allergic reaction in the patient
    b. The container is made of a substance that leaches into the medication
    c. There is no quantity of the contents listed on the container
    d. The drug is exposed to unsanitary conditions
    e. The patient writes the indication for the medication on their prescription bottle

41. Which of the following requirements must be met for a controlled substance prescription to be valid? Select ALL that apply.
    a. Must be manually signed if it is a paper or faxed prescription
    b. Must be issued for a legitimate medical purpose
    c. Must be prescribed in the usual course of medical treatment
    d. Must be issued to an individual practitioner for the purpose of general dispensing to patients
    e. Must be dated and signed on the fill date

42. According to the FDA, a drug is considered to be an orphan drug if it is for rare diseases or conditions that impact fewer than how many people in the U.S.?
    a. 10
    b. 500
    c. 200,000
    d. 1,000,000
    e. 2,000,000

43. Which of the following ingredients has special labeling requirements if it is included in a product?
    a. Gelatin
    b. FD&C Yellow No. 5
    c. High fructose corn syrup
    d. Sorbitol
    e. Xanthan gum

44. In which case(s) is it appropriate to receive a faxed prescription for a Schedule II controlled substance?

    I.   Patient is a resident of a long-term care facility (LTCF)

    II. Patient is enrolled in hospice program

    III. Medication is intended for home infusion therapy

    a. I only
    b. II only
    c. I and II
    d. II and III
    e. I, II, and III

45. What is the acronym of the voluntary reporting system for medication adverse events?
    a. VAERS
    b. FAERS
    c. ERSA
    d. MAERS
    e. AERS

46. Within how many days must a prescriber deliver a written prescription for a Schedule II controlled substance that was called in orally to be dispensed in an emergency situation?
    a. 3 days
    b. 5 days
    c. 7 days
    d. 14 days
    e. 15 days

47. A pharmacy intern wants to know where to find information on therapeutic equivalence between biologics. Which book contains this information?
    a. Red Book
    b. Purple Book
    c. Pink Book
    d. Orange Book
    e. Yellow Book

48. In which case(s) must an exact count be taken while performing a controlled substance inventory?

    I. It is a Schedule II controlled substance

    II. The bottle holds more than 1000 tablets or capsules

    III. Containers are sealed or unopened

    a. I only
    b. II only
    c. I and II
    d. II and III
    e. I, II, and III

49. The scheduling of controlled substances at the federal level is performed by the:
    a. Food and Drug Administration
    b. U.S. Attorney General
    c. Drug Enforcement Agency
    d. National Board of Pharmacy
    e. Drug Enforcement Administration

50. A manufacturer of a prescription-only drug wants to reclassify the drug as an over-the-counter (OTC) drug. What is one of the forms that may be submitted to the FDA when requesting reclassification of a prescription-only drug to an over-the-counter drug?
    a. Emergency Investigational New Drug Application (EIND)
    b. Investigational New Drug Application (IND)
    c. New Drug Application (NDA)
    d. Abbreviated New Drug Application (ANDA)
    e. Marketed New Drug Application (MNDA)

51. You are a pharmacist that suspects a fake controlled substance prescription was called in to your pharmacy. You use the numbers in the provided DEA to verify if it is a true DEA number. It is indeed not a true DEA number because the last number is incorrect. The DEA number is BS5927683. What would be the correct last digit of the DEA number if it was accurate?
    a. 1
    b. 2
    c. 4
    d. 5
    e. 6

52. Which of the following prescriptions would likely be out of the scope of practice for a dentist?
    a. Tylenol #3
    b. Amoxicillin
    c. Lorazepam
    d. Atorvastatin
    e. None of the above; dentists are not limited to scope of practice

53. Who is authorized to sign a DEA Form 222 at a community pharmacy?
    a. Any pharmacist
    b. Any pharmacist or technician
    c. Only the pharmacist-in-charge
    d. Only the pharmacist who signed the most recent application for renewal of the pharmacy's DEA registration
    e. The pharmacist who signed the most recent application for renewal of the pharmacy's DEA registration or someone authorized under a power of attorney

54. What types of patients are included in a Phase I clinical trial for drug development?
    a. Large group of non-human animals
    b. Small group of healthy participants without the disease condition
    c. Small group of participants with the disease condition
    d. Large group of healthy participants without the disease condition
    e. Large group of participants with the disease condition

55. A pharmacy may keep which of the following records at a central location other than the location registered with the DEA?
    a. Controlled substance inventories
    b. Controlled substance prescriptions
    c. Controlled substance shipping and financial records
    d. Copies of executed DEA Form 222 orders
    e. None of the above may be kept at a central location; all must be kept at the pharmacy

56. Acetaminophen with codeine (Tylenol #3) is classified under which controlled substance schedule?
    a. Schedule I
    b. Schedule II
    c. Schedule III
    d. Schedule IV
    e. Schedule V

57. A patient is admitted to a hospital and does not remember the names of the medications that she takes at home. The hospital pharmacist calls the patient's outpatient pharmacy to obtain a list of medications. Which of the following statements is true?
    a. This is a HIPAA violation unless the patient has given signed consent for the information to be given to the hospital
    b. This is a HIPAA violation unless the patient has given verbal consent for the information to be given to the hospital
    c. This is a HIPAA violation unless the patient has given written and verbal consent for the information to be given to the hospital
    d. This is not a HIPAA violation because HIPAA does not apply to patients being treated in a hospital setting
    e. This is not a HIPAA violation because the information is being given to the hospital for treatment purposes

58. A warning stating "Caution: Federal law prohibits the transfer of this drug to any person other than the patient for whom it was prescribed" is required on the label on which of the following prescriptions?
    a. Schedule II controlled substances only
    b. Schedule II–IV controlled substances only
    c. Schedule II–V controlled substances only
    d. Schedule III–V controlled substances only
    e. All prescriptions require this warning under federal law

59. Registering with the FDA as an outsourcing facility allows a pharmacy to:
    a. Compound sterile products without receiving patient-specific prescriptions
    b. Act as a mail order pharmacy with the ability to send medications to multiple states
    c. Process prescriptions and medication orders remotely for another pharmacy, but not dispense any medications
    d. Repackage medications so that they can be used at hospitals and other institutions
    e. Order drug products listed on the FDA drug shortage list at a discounted cost

60. In the event of a breach of unsecured protected health information (PHI) at a retail pharmacy affecting approximately 900 patients, who must be notified? Select ALL that apply.
    a. All nearby pharmacies
    b. Prominent local media outlets
    c. Affected patients
    d. All patients who use the pharmacy
    e. U.S. Secretary of Health and Human Services (HHS)

61. Standards and requirements for preparing sterile compounded drugs to ensure patient benefit and reduce risks such as contamination, infection, or incorrect dosing are outlined in which of the following?
    a. USP Chapter <503A>
    b. USP Chapter <503B>
    c. USP Chapter <795>
    d. USP Chapter <797>
    e. USP Chapter <800>

62. Which of the following is/are required to register with the Drug Enforcement Administration (DEA)? Select ALL that apply.
    a. A patient who receives a prescription for a controlled substance
    b. A manufacturer that manufactures controlled substances
    c. A pharmacy that dispenses controlled substances
    d. A physician who prescribes controlled substances
    e. A pharmacist who dispenses controlled substances

63. Which of the following medications requires Risk Evaluation and Mitigation Strategy (REMS) monitoring?
    a. Hydromorphone (Dilaudid)
    b. Clozapine (Clozaril)
    c. Fluoxetine (Prozac)
    d. Zolpidem (Ambien)
    e. Metformin (Glucophage)

64. A DEA Form 41 is used to document which of the following?
    a. Purchasing of controlled substances from a manufacturer
    b. Transfer of controlled substances to a reverse distributor
    c. On-site destruction of controlled substances
    d. Significant loss or theft of controlled substances
    e. None of the above

65. What act set the requirement for tamper-evident packaging for some over-the-counter products in order to avoid risk of contamination?
    a. Safe Drug Packaging Act
    b. Federal Anti-Tampering Act
    c. Drug Contamination Prevention Act
    d. Federal Anti-Contamination Act
    e. Tamper-Evident Packaging Act

66. Drugs that have a high potential for abuse and severe potential for dependence with no currently accepted medical use in the U.S. are classified as:
    a. Schedule I
    b. Schedule II
    c. Schedule III
    d. Schedule IV
    e. None of the above

67. Which of the following is NOT required to be included on a manufacturer's container of an over-the-counter (OTC) medication?
    a. Warnings
    b. Inactive ingredients
    c. Poison Control Center phone number
    d. Purpose
    e. Directions

68. A nursing home patient who is prescribed an estrogen-containing product must be given a Patient Package Insert (PPI):
    a. Prior to the first administration only
    b. Prior to the first administration and every 30 days thereafter
    c. Prior to the first administration and every 60 days thereafter
    d. Only when requested by the patient
    e. None of the above

69. For how long is a DEA registration for possession of controlled substances valid?
    a. 12 months
    b. 24 months
    c. 36 months
    d. 48 months
    e. 60 months

70. Which of the following statements is/are true regarding DEA Form 222?

    I.   Executed copies of DEA Form 222 must be maintained separately from all other records.

    II. A defective DEA Form 222 may be corrected and reused.

    III. On the DEA Form 222, only 1 item may be entered on each numbered line.

    a. I only
    b. II only
    c. I and III only
    d. II and III only
    e. I, II, and III

71. An independent community pharmacy wants to start offering refill reminders to patients in the form of a postcard mailed to the patient's house. The fee for this service would be $2 per month. Which of the following is true regarding this service?
    a. This service cannot be provided because it creates a HIPAA violation
    b. Signed authorization would be required from each patient, as this is considered use of protected health information (PHI) for marketing purposes
    c. This service does not violate HIPAA, but patients cannot be charged a fee for refill reminders
    d. This service does not violate HIPAA, but the reminders must be transmitted electronically
    e. There are no barriers to offering this service and the pharmacy can proceed as planned

72. The expiration date on a bottle of metformin purchased from a manufacturer by a pharmacy is listed as 03/22. What is the expiration date of the drug?
    a. March 1, 2022
    b. March 19, 2022
    c. March 30, 2022
    d. March 31, 2022
    e. None of the above

73. A prospective drug utilization review (DUR) consists of reviewing all of the following aspects of a prescription EXCEPT for:
    a. Underutilization
    b. Therapeutic duplication
    c. Compliance with prescription labeling
    d. Appropriate dosing and regimen
    e. Drug interactions

74. Which of the following statements is required on an over-the-counter (OTC) package of acetaminophen tablets under the Federal Hazardous Substances Act?
    a. "Keep out of the reach of children"
    b. "Consult a doctor before use"
    c. "Do not use if pregnant or breastfeeding"
    d. "Prescription not required"
    e. "For adult use only"

75. A pharmacy dispenses and distributes a total of 50,000 doses of controlled substances in a 12-month period. How many doses is the pharmacy able to transfer to another pharmacy without registering as a distributor?
    a. 500 doses
    b. 1,000 doses
    c. 2,500 doses
    d. 5,000 doses
    e. 10,000 doses

76. The Occupational and Safety Health Administration (OSHA) requires that pharmacies do which of the following?
    a. Provide patients with information regarding the safe handling of hazardous medications
    b. Provide patients with Safety Data Sheets for hazardous medications
    c. Include the word "caution" or "warning" on labels for all hazardous medications
    d. Train all of their employees on the hazards of chemicals and on the protective measures they should take
    e. None of the above

77. The Poison Prevention Packaging Act (PPPA), which requires child-resistant containers for prescription and certain non-prescription drugs (with some exceptions), is administered by the:
    a. Food and Drug Administration
    b. Consumer Product Safety Commission
    c. Federal Trade Commission
    d. Centers for Medicare and Medicaid Services
    e. Occupational and Safety Health Administration

78. A pharmacy orders bulk bottles of ibuprofen and compounds ibuprofen suppositories. These suppositories are sold to other pharmacies that need to fill prescriptions but do not have the ability to make them. Which of the following terms best describes this practice?
    a. Compounding
    b. Dispensing
    c. Bulk compounding
    d. Manufacturing
    e. Outsourcing

79. Which of the following is true regarding the purchasing and selling of prescription drug samples?
    a. Drug samples may be purchased by a community pharmacy from a drug company and sold to patients at a standard price set by the FDA
    b. Drug samples may be purchased by a community pharmacy but must be given to patients free of charge
    c. Drug samples may only be given to a patient at a community pharmacy if the patient already has a prescription for the same medication
    d. Drug samples may be given to a pharmacy owned by a charitable organization and sold to patients at a reduced cost if the facility provides care to indigent or low-income patients
    e. Drug samples may be given to a pharmacy which is owned by a charitable organization that provides care to indigent or low-income patients, but must be given to patients free of charge

80. Which of the following is a valid method of ordering Schedule III medications from a supplier to restock a pharmacy's bulk medication supply?
    a. Mailing a hard copy of DEA Form 222 to the supplier
    b. Mailing a hard copy of DEA Form 224 to the supplier
    c. Faxing a copy of DEA Form 222 to the supplier
    d. Faxing a copy of DEA Form 224 to the supplier
    e. Sending an online order to the supplier with no additional form sent

81. Which of the following products is NOT required to be in tamper-evident packaging for retail sale?
    a. Acetaminophen tablets
    b. Children's diphenhydramine liquid
    c. Aspirin tablets
    d. Benzocaine/menthol lozenges
    e. Infant simethicone drops

82. A pharmacist may call a prescriber and receive verbal permission to change all of the following on a Schedule II prescription EXCEPT:
    a. Quantity
    b. Directions for use
    c. Drug name
    d. Drug strength
    e. Dosage form

83. A patient requests a copy of her prescription records from a community pharmacy. Within what time period must the pharmacy provide this information?
    a. 24 hours
    b. 3 days
    c. 7 days
    d. 10 days
    e. 30 days

84. Which of the following drugs has a REMS program due to a high frequency of birth defects?
    a. Lisinopril
    b. Thalidomide
    c. Zyprexa
    d. Atorvastatin
    e. Levothyroxine

85. Which law requires new drugs to be proven as safe and effective before approval?
    a. Poison Prevention Packaging Act
    b. Durham-Humphrey Amendment
    c. Kefauver-Harris Amendment
    d. Prescription Drug Marketing Act
    e. Drug Quality and Security Act

86. Anabolic steroids are classified under which controlled substance schedule under federal law?
    a. Schedule I
    b. Schedule II
    c. Schedule III
    d. Schedule IV
    e. Schedule V

87. Which act or amendment created the separation of drugs into two different categories, prescription (legend) and over-the-counter?
    a. Kefauver-Harris Amendment
    b. Omnibus Reconciliation Act
    c. Hatch-Waxman Amendment
    d. Durham-Humphrey Amendment
    e. Robinson-Patman Act

88. A patient picks up a prescription for Xarelto at a community pharmacy, but returns later in the day concerned that the prescription was filled with generic rivaroxaban. The pharmacist explains that the prescription was filled with the generic form of the medication because it was cheaper than using the brand name product. The patient asks if the generic will work as well as the brand name product. According to the pharmacist's drug reference, the two products have an FDA equivalency rating of AB. What is the proper interpretation of this code?
    a. The products are not bioequivalent, and the prescription should be filled only with brand name Xarelto
    b. The products have not been studied to determine bioequivalence, so a determination cannot be made
    c. The products have no known or suspected bioequivalence issues and are interchangeable
    d. The products may have actual or potential bioequivalence issues, but there is adequate evidence to use them interchangeably
    e. The code AB alone does not provide enough information to determine bioequivalence

89. DEA registration is NOT required for which of the following situations? Select ALL that apply.
    a. A nurse who is working in a physician's office where controlled substances are prescribed
    b. A pharmacist who regularly dispenses controlled substances at a community pharmacy
    c. A physician who occasionally prescribes controlled substances at a private clinic
    d. A patient who picks up a prescription for a newly prescribed controlled substance
    e. A pharmacy dispensing controlled substances

90. A drug manufacturer finds that bottles labeled "loratadine 10mg tablets" actually contain 5mg tablets, and issues a recall of the affected lot. Which of the following is true of this product?
    a. It is adulterated
    b. It is misbranded
    c. It is contaminated
    d. It is both adulterated and misbranded
    e. None of the above

91. A physician writes a prescription for ibuprofen 800mg tablets for a patient with rheumatoid arthritis. On the prescription, the physician adds a note that says, "please place this prescription and all future prescriptions in easy-open containers, as the patient is unable to open child-resistant bottles." Which of the following is true regarding this request?
    a. It is not valid because providers do not have the authority to request special packaging on a patient's behalf
    b. It is not valid because ibuprofen is not on the list of drugs exempt from the child-resistant packaging requirement under the Poison Prevention Packaging Act
    c. It is not valid because the provider must submit a separate signed form to make this request
    d. The ibuprofen can be dispensed in an easy-open container, but the blanket request to provide easy-open caps on all future prescriptions is not valid because only the patient can make such a request
    e. It is valid and a note should be made on the patient's profile to use easy-open containers on all prescriptions in the future

92. Which of the following would NOT be considered a potential part of a Risk Evaluation and Mitigation Strategy (REMS) program?
    a. Requiring special certification for pharmacies, practitioners, or health care settings that dispense a drug
    b. Requiring laboratory testing to ensure safe use of a drug
    c. Performing a financial assessment to ensure that a patient can afford a drug for the duration of treatment
    d. Providing a medication guide to patients which includes information about a drug
    e. Requiring that a patient enroll in a registry when they begin taking a drug

93. Retail containers of chewable low-dose 81mg aspirin (1.25 grain) must have special warnings for use in children including a warning regarding Reye's syndrome, and cannot contain more than:
    a. 10 tablets
    b. 30 tablets
    c. 36 tablets
    d. 48 tablets
    e. 60 tablets

94. Which of these is a valid DEA registration number for a mid-level practitioner?
    a. M11496023
    b. MT1200980
    c. CR5624112
    d. MM7411222
    e. BL115231

95. The FDA may require a medication guide be issued with certain prescriptions for which reason(s)? Select ALL that apply.
    a. When a drug has serious risks relative to benefits
    b. When patient adherence is crucial
    c. When the patient is a resident of a nursing home or other institution
    d. When drug information can prevent serious adverse effects
    e. When a pharmacist is unavailable to provide counseling on a new prescription

96. What act set the requirement that patients must be offered counseling on dispensed medications?
    a. OSHA 90
    b. DATA 90
    c. HCFA 90
    d. OPDP 90
    e. OBRA 90

97. Which of the following is/are NOT required to be packaged in a child-resistant container? Select ALL that apply.
    a. A container of 30 sublingual nitroglycerin tablets
    b. A methylprednisolone dose pack containing 21 tablets that are 4mg each
    c. A container of 100 aspirin tablets
    d. A prednisone dose pack containing 21 tablets that are 10mg each
    e. An albuterol inhaler

98. Prescription records must be kept for a minimum of _____ based on federal law.
    a. 1 year
    b. 2 years
    c. 3 years
    d. 4 years
    e. 5 years

99. A pharmacist dispenses a prescription for aripiprazole at an outpatient pharmacy. When is a medication guide required?
    a. Only for the first dispensing
    b. Every time the drug is filled, including refills
    c. Only if the patient requests
    d. The pharmacist may determine if a medication guide is necessary
    e. A medication guide is not required

100. To comply with Centers for Medicare and Medicaid Services (CMS) requirements, how often must a pharmacist conduct a drug regimen review for long-term care patients?
    a. At least once a week
    b. At least once a month
    c. At least once every 60 days
    d. At least once every 6 months
    e. Annually

Washington MPJE Questions

1. Which of the following is/are true regarding a pharmacist prescribing controlled substances while working under a collaborative drug therapy agreement (CDTA)? Select ALL that apply.
    a. The pharmacist must have his or her own DEA number
    b. The scope of the CDTA must permit the prescribing of controlled substances
    c. Any pharmacist licensed in the state of Washington may prescribe controlled substances
    d. The pharmacist may use the authorizing prescriber's DEA number
    e. Pharmacists are not allowed to prescribe controlled substances, even under a CDTA

2. A drug has been changed from non-controlled to controlled substance status. When does a pharmacy need to conduct an inventory of controlled substances?
    a. On the effective date when the drug is added to the controlled substance schedule
    b. One week before the drug is added to the controlled substance schedule
    c. Within one week after the drug is added to the controlled substance schedule
    d. Within one month after the drug is added to the controlled substance schedule
    e. Conducting controlled substance inventory is not required in this case

3. Who is in charge of the storage, distribution, and control of approved investigational drugs used in an institution?
   a. Registered pharmacist
   b. Pharmacy technician
   c. Director of pharmacy or their designee
   d. Principal investigator
   e. Pharmacist manager

4. Gabapentin is not federally classified as a controlled substance. Which of the following is/are true regarding gabapentin in Washington?

   I. Gabapentin is not classified as a controlled substance in Washington.

   II. Gabapentin prescription information must be transmitted to the prescription monitoring program (PMP).

   III. Gabapentin has been classified as a Schedule V controlled substance by the commission.

   a. I only
   b. I and II only
   c. I and III only
   d. II and III only
   e. I, II, and III

5. Central fill shared pharmacy services may be provided at off-site locations. When the services performed include prescription fulfillment or processing, the pharmacy must comply with which of the following? Select ALL that apply.
   a. The originating pharmacy must have written policies and procedures outlining the off-site pharmacy services to be provided by the central fill pharmacy
   b. The off-site pharmacy must retain records for dispensing and must notify the originating pharmacy within 1 business day of any services provided
   c. The parties must share a secure real-time database or utilize other secure technology
   d. The originating pharmacy must transfer prescriptions to the off-site pharmacy prior to fulfillment
   e. The off-site pharmacy must register as a wholesale pharmacy

6. Which of the following is/are true when the governor issues an emergency proclamation and pharmacies may provide emergency prescription medications?

    I. A pharmacist can provide up to a 30-day supply for non-controlled prescriptions

    II. A pharmacist can provide up to a 7-day supply for Schedule III, IV, and V controlled substance prescriptions

    III. A pharmacist can dispense a one-time emergency refill for an expired prescription

      a. I only
      b. II only
      c. III only
      d. I and II only
      e. I, II, and III

7. Which of the following statements is/are true regarding pharmacies storing, dispensing, and delivering drugs to patients without a pharmacist on-site?

    I. The pharmacy is required to have adequate visual surveillance of the full pharmacy and retain a high-quality recording for a minimum of one year

    II. The responsible pharmacy manager must conduct an inspection of the off-site pharmacy biennially

    III. A pharmacist must be capable of being on-site at the pharmacy within three hours if an emergency arises

    IV. The pharmacy is required to have a visual and audio communication system used to counsel and interact with each patient or patient's caregiver

      a. I only
      b. II only
      c. I and II
      d. III and IV
      e. I, II, III, and IV

8. Which of the following is/are required on the label for a prepackaged medication in an emergency department when pharmacy services are unavailable? Select ALL that apply.
    I. Drug name
    II. Complete directions for use
    III. Expiration date
    IV. Lot number
    V. Patient name

9. Which of the following is/are true regarding transferring a prescription?

    I. Sufficient information needs to be exchanged to maintain an auditable trail

    II. Pharmacies sharing a secure real-time database are not required to transfer prescription information for dispensing

    III. Prescriptions must be transferred by electronic means or facsimile except in emergency situations

    a. I only
    b. II only
    c. I and II only
    d. I and III only
    e. I, II, and III

10. All of the following are true regarding a pharmacy's electronic systems for patient medication records, prescriptions, chart orders, and controlled substance records EXCEPT:
    a. A pharmacy shall use an electronic record-keeping system to store patient information, prescription information, and other relevant information for patient care
    b. The electronic system must have security features to protect confidentiality of records
    c. The electronic system must be capable of real-time retrieval of information pertaining to ordering, verification, and processing of prescriptions
    d. The pharmacy must have policies and procedures for system downtime
    e. A retail pharmacy may opt out of using electronic record-keeping systems with permission from the Board.

11. How are ephedrine products classified by the commission?
    a. Over-the-counter drugs
    b. Legend drugs
    c. Schedule III drugs
    d. Schedule IV drugs
    e. The commission does not explicitly state a classification for ephedrine products

12. Which of the following statements is/are true for a pharmacist license that has been expired for three years or more when the pharmacist has not been in practice in another state?

    I.   The pharmacist must service an internship of 300 hours

    II. The pharmacist must pass the jurisprudence exam (MPJE)

    III. The pharmacist must pass the licensure exam (NAPLEX)

    a. I only
    b. II only
    c. II and III only
    d. I and II only
    e. I, II, and III

13. Which of the following statements is/are true?

    I.   A corporation may advertise controlled substances for sale to the general public

    II. Controlled substances may be physically displayed to the public

    III. Controlled substances may not be physically displayed to the public

    a. I only
    b. I and II only
    c. I and III only
    d. II only
    e. III only

14. Which of the following is a legend (prescription only) drug according to the board of pharmacy?
    a. Theodrine tablet (25mg ephedrine HCl)
    b. Quelidrine (5mg ephedrine HCl)
    c. Primatene tablet (24mg ephedrine HCl)
    d. All of the above
    e. None of the above

15. Which of the following statements is true regarding the retail sale of dextromethorphan?
    a. It is unlawful to sell a finished drug product containing any quantity of dextromethorphan to a person less than 21 years old
    b. A person making a retail sale of a finished product containing dextromethorphan must obtain proof of age from the purchaser before completing the sale, unless the purchaser's outward appearance appears to be 25 years of age or older
    c. It is unlawful to sell a finished drug product containing any quantity of dextromethorphan to a person less than 18 years of age
    d. Both (b) and (c)
    e. None of the above

16. Pharmacies serving hospitals and long-term care facilities may accept drug returns for future dispensing based on which of the following criteria?
    a. Chain of custody is maintained and product integrity is ensured
    b. The drug must be in its original sealed package
    c. The drug must be in unit dose packaging
    d. The drug must be in either an original sealed package or unit dose packaging
    e. The return of any drugs is prohibited

17. A patient complains that her medication bottles are too difficult to open because of her arthritis. Who can give authorization to dispense prescriptions in containers that are not child-resistant (i.e., easy open caps)? Select ALL that apply.
    a. The prescriber
    b. The patient
    c. The patient's representative
    d. The pharmacist
    e. The pharmacist manager

18. What is the maximum supply of prepackaged medication that can be dispensed in an emergency department when pharmacy services are unavailable?
    a. 24 hours
    b. 36 hours
    c. 48 hours
    d. 72 hours
    e. 96 hours

19. How many hours of acquired immunodeficiency syndrome (AIDS) education is required for a pharmacist to become licensed in Washington state?
    a. 1 hour
    b. 2 hours
    c. 5 hours
    d. 7 hours
    e. 10 hours

20. All of the following are minimum requirements for a pharmacy EXCEPT:
    a. The facility is constructed and equipped with adequate security
    b. A pharmacy manager shall be named within 30 days of opening a pharmacy
    c. The facility shall create policies on the purchasing, ordering, compounding, delivery, and dispensing of drugs
    d. The facility shall submit to the commission a utilization plan for pharmacy technicians and pharmacy assistants
    e. Each dispensed prescription must bear a complete and accurate label

21. Which of the following is/are true regarding pharmacist license renewal?

    I. 30 hours of continuing education is required over the span of two years

    II. Pharmacist license renewal is annual

    III. The license expires on the pharmacist's birthdate

    a. I only
    b. II only
    c. I and II only
    d. I and III only
    e. I, II, and III

22. What criteria must be met for a pharmacist to become a preceptor?

    I.   Practice pharmacy for at least 12 months

    II.   Submit an application through the Washington State Department of Health

    III.   There is no special criteria for a pharmacist to hold a preceptor certification

    a. I only
    b. II only
    c. III only
    d. I and II only
    e. I, II, and III

23. Who may receive prescription monitoring program (PMP) information from the department? Select ALL that apply.
    a. Any public or private entity for statistical, research, or educational purposes
    b. Washington state hospital association's coordinated quality improvement program (CQIP)
    c. A patient's personal representative
    d. Federal law enforcement official
    e. A medical examiner

24. Which of the following statements is/are true about refilling a prescription when the prescriber is unavailable for refill authorization? Select ALL that apply.
    a. The prescription refill cannot be for a controlled drug
    b. The refill cannot exceed a 72-hour supply
    c. The prescriber must be notified within one business day
    d. Refills without prescriber authorization are prohibited
    e. A pharmacist may dispense up to a 30-day supply

25. How many times can a prescription for a Schedule II controlled substance be refilled?
    a. 0
    b. 1
    c. 2
    d. 3
    e. 4

26. Pharmacy assistants may perform which of the following under the supervision of a licensed pharmacist?

    I. Typing of prescription labels

    II. Stocking

    III. Refilling prescriptions

    a. I only
    b. III only
    c. I and II only
    d. II and III only
    e. I, II, and III

27. A long-term care pharmacy using shared pharmacy service is unable to provide a prescription to a patient. A secondary supplying pharmacy is able to provide the first dose to meet the patient's immediate need. What must the pharmacies do in this situation?
    a. The outsourcing pharmacy must transfer the original prescription and all refills to the supplying pharmacy
    b. The outsourcing pharmacy must transfer the original prescription to the supplying pharmacy but can retain information for the corresponding refills
    c. The outsourcing pharmacy must fully transfer the prescription to the supplying pharmacy
    d. The supplying pharmacy may dispense the first dose without fully transferring the prescription
    e. The supplying pharmacy must contact the prescriber to obtain a new prescription

28. When must a pharmacy pay the original licensing fee for pharmacies? Select ALL that apply.
    a. Prior to opening a new pharmacy
    b. An existing pharmacy's location changes
    c. An existing pharmacy's ownership changes
    d. An existing pharmacy's business structure changes (ex: sole proprietorship to corporation)
    e. An existing pharmacy is remodeled

29. Which of the following statements is/are true regarding drug price advertising by a pharmacy?

    I.   The advertising is directed towards providing consumers with drug price information

    II.   The advertising promotes the use of the prescription drug to the public

    III.   The advertising must include the drug's strength

    a. I only
    b. II only
    c. I and II only
    d. I and III only
    e. I, II, and III

30. A prescription for a Schedule V controlled substance may not be filled more than _____ from date of issue or refilled more than _____.
    a. 90 days; 1 time
    b. 90 days; 5 times
    c. 6 months; 1 time
    d. 6 months; 5 times
    e. 12 months; 12 times

31. In which of the following situations is a prescription considered invalid?

    I.   The prescription shows evidence of alteration

    II.   A controlled substance prescription is missing directions for use

    III.   The prescription is for a controlled substance and the dispense date is 60 days from the date of issue

    a. I only
    b. II only
    c. I and II only
    d. II and III only
    e. I, II, and III

32. In an extended care facility, emergency kits shall be accessible to:
    a. Licensed nurses
    b. Medical Assistants
    c. Caregivers
    d. Patients
    e. Patient service representatives

33. To transfer an original prescription for a non-controlled drug for the purpose of refill dispensing, which of the following requirements must be met?

    I. Prescriptions must be transferred by electronic means or facsimile

    II. Sufficient information needs to be exchanged in the transfer of a prescription to maintain an auditable trail, as well as all elements of a valid prescription

    III. Pharmacies sharing a secure real-time database must also transfer prescription information for dispensing

    a. I only
    b. I and II only
    c. I and III only
    d. II and III only
    e. I, II, and III

34. All the following are true regarding drug samples EXCEPT:
    a. A retail pharmacy may distribute drug samples
    b. A dental practice may distribute drug samples
    c. A surgical center may distribute drug samples
    d. A manufacturer may distribute drug samples
    e. A hospital may distribute drug samples

35. What information is required on hospital inpatient prescription labels? Select ALL that apply.
    a. Drug name (generic and/or trade)
    b. Auxiliary labels listing storage requirements
    c. Drug strength
    d. Patient name
    e. Prescriber name

36. How long is a prescription for a non-controlled drug valid?
    a. 90 days
    b. 6 months
    c. 12 months
    d. 2 years
    e. No expiration date exists

37. What is the minimum retention period for original prescriptions and refill records?
    a. 1 year
    b. 2 years
    c. 3 years
    d. 4 years
    e. 5 years

38. Which of the following is true regarding controlled substance recordkeeping?
    a. Controlled substance records must be kept for five years
    b. Records for Schedule II controlled substances can be maintained separately from or together with controlled substance records
    c. A pharmacy that operates without a pharmacist on-site must maintain a perpetual inventory
    d. Controlled substance inventory must be conducted annually
    e. Invoices for controlled substances only need to be kept for one year

39. A partial fill of a Schedule II controlled substance is permitted under which circumstance(s)? Select ALL that apply.
    a. If requested by the practitioner
    b. If requested by the patient
    c. If the pharmacist determines quantity is too high
    d. If the total quantity requested in all partial fillings does not exceed the quantity prescribed
    e. If the total quantity requested exceeds the quantity prescribed

40. Which of the following is required on a prescription for a non-controlled drug?
    a. Patient's address
    b. Prescriber's name
    c. Prescriber's DEA number
    d. Patient's allergies
    e. Patient's phone number

41. How long is a prescription for a Schedule II controlled substance valid?
    a. 60 days
    b. 90 days
    c. 6 months
    d. 12 months
    e. 1 year

42. A physician is sending an electronic prescription for hydrocodone-acetaminophen to the pharmacy. All of the following are required on the prescription EXCEPT:
    a. Prescriber's electronic signature
    b. Prescriber's DEA number
    c. Prescriber's address
    d. Patient's address
    e. Patient's allergies

43. For which indication(s) may a Schedule II stimulant be prescribed? Select ALL that apply.
    a. Shift work disorders
    b. Binge eating disorders
    c. Drug-induced brain dysfunction
    d. Narcolepsy
    e. Weight loss

44. Which of the following is/are required on the label of prepackaged medications? Select ALL that apply.
    a. Drug name
    b. Drug strength
    c. Expiration date
    d. Manufacturer's name and lot number (if not maintained in a separate record)
    e. Identity of pharmacist or provider responsible for prepackaging (if not maintained in a separate record)

45. All of the following are required on an outpatient prescription label EXCEPT:
    a. Prescriber's address
    b. Name of prescriber
    c. Complete directions for use
    d. Name of drug
    e. Number of refills remaining, if any

46. How many years must a pharmaceutical manufacturer, wholesaler, pharmacy, or practitioner retain invoices to account for the receipt of legend drugs?
    a. 2 years
    b. 3 years
    c. 5 years
    d. 10 years
    e. There is no requirement to maintain invoices

47. Which of the following can be a function of the pharmacy technician?
    a. Consult with a prescriber regarding a patient's prescription
    b. Interpret data in a patient medication record
    c. Patient counseling
    d. Enter a prescription into the pharmacy computer
    e. Accept call-in prescriptions from a physician's office

48. All of the following are true regarding poison sales EXCEPT:
    a. When purchasing poisons, the purchaser must present identification that contains the purchaser's photograph and signature
    b. Both the purchaser and the seller must sign the poison register entry
    c. The seller must determine that the poison will be used for a lawful purpose
    d. The purchaser can refuse to disclose why the poison is being purchased
    e. The seller must determine that the purchaser's identification matches the purchaser's representations

49. What is the maximum pharmacist to technician ratio in a pharmacy?
    a. 1:1
    b. 1:2
    c. 1:3
    d. 1:4
    e. As determined by the pharmacy manager

50. For a qualifying patient taking medical marijuana, what is the maximum number of marijuana plants that may be grown or located in any one housing unit?
    a. 10
    b. 15
    c. 20
    d. 25
    e. 30

51. Which of the following is/are true concerning transferring prescriptions to another pharmacy? Select ALL that apply.
    a. A pharmacist must transfer all prescriptions
    b. A pharmacist must transfer all controlled prescriptions
    c. A pharmacy technician, under a pharmacist's supervision, may transfer controlled prescriptions by fax
    d. A pharmacy technician, under a pharmacist's supervision, may transfer noncontrolled prescriptions by fax
    e. A pharmacy technician, under a pharmacist's supervision, may transfer noncontrolled prescriptions verbally over the phone

52. Which of the following statements is/are true regarding 'The Washington Death with Dignity Act'?

    I. A valid request for medication to end the patient's life needs to be signed and dated by the patient and 2 witnesses

    II. The attending physician and consulting physician determine the patient is suffering from a terminal disease, is a resident of Washington State, and is competent

    III. An adult who makes a written request for medication to end his or her life is doing so based on an informed decision

    a. I only
    b. II only
    c. III only
    d. II and III only
    e. I, II, and III

53. A Medicare-approved dialysis center may sell, deliver, or dispense to its dialysis patients all of the following legend drugs, if prescribed by a physician, EXCEPT:
    a. Sterile heparin, 1000 units/mL in vials
    b. Sterile potassium chloride 2 mEq/mL for injection
    c. Commercially available dialysate
    d. Sterile sodium chloride, 0.9% for injection in containers of not less than 150ml
    e. Epoetin alfa (Epogen) in vials

54. The prescription monitoring program was designed for which of the following purposes?
    a. To detect and prevent prescription drug abuse
    b. To improve health care quality and effectiveness
    c. To reduce duplicative prescribing and overprescribing of controlled substances
    d. To improve controlled substance prescribing practices
    e. All of the above

55. When submitting a drug prescription to the prescription monitoring program (PMP), which of the following is/are required? Select ALL that apply.
    a. Patient identifier
    b. Drug dispensed
    c. Prescriber
    d. Dispenser
    e. Quantity dispensed

56. All of the following are requirements for pharmacy technician certification EXCEPT:
    a. Applicant must be at least 18 years old and hold a high school diploma or GED
    b. Applicant must provide proof of completing 8 hours of guided study of Washington state and federal pharmacy law
    c. Applicant must provide proof of successful completion of a commission-approved pharmacy technician program
    d. Applicant must pass a national certification examination within 1 year of completing their training program and applying for certification
    e. Applicant must provide a letter of recommendation from their employer

57. A temporary permit to practice pharmacy is issued to an applicant that meets what criteria? Select ALL that apply.
    a. Holds an unrestricted active license by examination in another state which participates in the license transfer or reciprocity process
    b. Has completed a Washington application for pharmacist license by transfer or reciprocity
    c. Has passed the Washington state jurisprudence exam
    d. Has submitted pharmacist license application fees
    e. Does not have a criminal record in Washington

58. Which of the following is/are true regarding pharmacist licenses in Washington?

    I.   A copy of each pharmacist's license must be on display for the public

    II.   Pharmacists who work in several locations should have a copy of their license for each location

    III.   The address on the pharmacy license cannot be obscured

    a. I only
    b. III only
    c. I and II only
    d. II and III only
    e. I, II, and III

59. As part of their continuing pharmacy education (CPE) requirements, pharmacists must complete a one-time training in which of these topics?
    a. Suicide prevention
    b. Antibiotic stewardship
    c. Naloxone training
    d. Pain management
    e. Human trafficking

60. The prescription monitoring program monitors the prescribing and dispensing of which drugs? Select ALL that apply.
    a. Schedule II controlled substances
    b. Schedule III controlled substances
    c. Schedule IV controlled substances
    d. Schedule V controlled substances
    e. Pseudoephedrine

61. What must a pharmacy do when there is a significant loss of controlled substances?
    a. Complete DEA form 106 and transmit to federal authorities only
    b. Complete DEA form 106 and transmit to the commission only
    c. Complete DEA form 106 and transmit two copies to federal authorities and transmit one copy to the commission
    d. Document the loss in biennial inventory and keep on file for 2 years
    e. There is no commission-approved protocol for significant loss

62. Which of the following statements is/are true about medical marijuana?

    I. The lawful possession of medical marijuana cannot result in forfeiture or seizure of property

    II. A qualifying patient needs to be entered into the medical marijuana authorization database

    III. A qualifying patient needs to hold a valid recognition card for possessing medical marijuana

    a. I only
    b. II only
    c. II and III only
    d. I and II only
    e. I, II, and III

63. How long must a patient's record be maintained by the pharmacy?
    a. 1 year
    b. 2 years
    c. 3 years
    d. 4 years
    e. 5 years

64. A pharmacy may fill a Schedule II narcotic substance prescription faxed by which location(s)? Select ALL that apply.
    a. Long-term care facility
    b. Retail pharmacy
    c. Hospice program
    d. Outpatient clinic pharmacy
    e. Hospital

65. How many pharmacists serve on the Washington Board of Pharmacy?
    a. 4 pharmacists
    b. 6 pharmacists
    c. 10 pharmacists
    d. 15 pharmacists
    e. 20 pharmacists

66. How many continuing pharmacy education contact hours are required for pharmacists every two years?
    a. 10 hours
    b. 15 hours
    c. 20 hours
    d. 30 hours
    e. There is no CPE requirement

67. Which of the following is true regarding picking up a controlled prescription?
    a. Only the patient listed on the prescription may pick up a controlled prescription
    b. The name of person picking up or dropping off a controlled prescription must always be verified by valid photographic identification
    c. The name of person picking up or dropping off a controlled prescription must be verified by valid photographic identification when practicable
    d. A prescriber may assign an agent to pick up a controlled prescription for a patient
    e. There are no current laws that mention picking up a controlled substance

68. Prescriptions for legend drugs are NOT allowed from which out-of-state prescriber?
    a. Physicians (MD)
    b. Dentists (DMD, DDS)
    c. Advanced registered nurse practitioners (ARNP)
    d. Optometrists (OD)
    e. Veterinarians (DVM)

69. Which of the following is/are true regarding pharmacy self-inspection? Select ALL that apply.
    a. A pharmacy self-inspection is completed every two years
    b. A pharmacy self-inspection is completed by a pharmacy manager (or equivalent)
    c. A pharmacy self-inspection is completed on worksheets provided by the commission
    d. If the pharmacy manager changes, a self-inspection must be completed by the new pharmacy manager within 30 days
    e. The pharmacy self-inspection worksheet must be maintained in the pharmacy for 5 years

70. Which of the following is/are true regarding electronic methamphetamine precursor tracking?

  I.   The signature must be captured electronically

  II. The purchaser's full name must be entered into the system as it appears on the photo identification that they provide

  III. If the tracking system is unavailable, a sale cannot be made

  a. I only
  b. II only
  c. III only
  d. II and III only
  e. I, II, and III

71. Which of the following statements is/are true regarding patient counseling?

  I.   Patient counseling can be performed by a pharmacy technician

  II. Counseling must be offered when filling a new prescription

  III. Counseling must be offered when refilling a prescription

  a. I only
  b. II only
  c. III only
  d. II and III only
  e. I, II, and III

72. When can a medication be dispensed in a container that is NOT child-resistant? Select ALL that apply.
  a. All medications must be dispensed in a child-resistant container
  b. When a patient requests an easy open container
  c. When a patient's representative requests an easy open container
  d. When a prescriber requests an easy open container
  e. When a pharmacist uses clinical judgement in providing an easy open container (ex. Arthritis medication)

73. Whenever a pharmacy closes, the owner is to notify the commission no later than how many days prior to the anticipated closing date?
    a. 2 days
    b. 5 days
    c. 15 days
    d. 20 days
    e. 30 days

74. In which of the following incidences may a pharmacist make an adaptation to a prescription with patient consent? Select ALL that apply.
    a. Changing the dosage form from tablet to capsule
    b. Changing the quantity on the prescription to match a commercially available package size
    c. Changing a generic drug to an alternative drug as long as it is in the same drug class
    d. Changing a 20mg tablet to two 10mg tablets
    e. Changing a drug to a different, lower cost drug indicated for certain diseases

75. A pharmacist may substitute a drug product or a biologic product according to a facility formulary if which of the following are met? Select ALL that apply.
    a. An outside facility prescribed the drug or biologic product to be substituted
    b. The formulary was composed by non-pharmacist prescribers only
    c. The formulary was readily retrievable by the pharmacist
    d. The formulary was created by an interdisciplinary team
    e. The institutional facility prescribed the drug or biologic product to be substituted

76. Which of the following is/are true regarding the prescription monitoring program (PMP) integration mandate? Select ALL that apply.
    a. A facility must submit a waiver to forego transmitting data to the PMP
    b. Internet speed could be an exceptional circumstance that a facility may use to waive the PMP mandate
    c. A practice generating less than 500 prescriptions for Schedule II-V drugs can apply for a PMP mandate waiver
    d. Upon the granting of a PMP waiver, a facility is exempt from the prescription monitoring program integration mandate for the calendar year
    e. A facility may submit up to three annual attestations in circumstance including economic hardship

77. Synthetic cannabinoids are listed under what controlled substance schedule?
    a. Schedule I
    b. Schedule II
    c. Schedule III
    d. Schedule IV
    e. Schedule V

78. When permanently closing a pharmacy, the Pharmacy Quality Assurance Commission must be notified no later than how many days prior to closing?
    a. 15 days prior
    b. 30 days prior
    c. 45 days prior
    d. 60 days prior
    e. 90 days prior

79. How many continuing pharmacy education contact hours are required for pharmacy technicians every two years?
    a. 10 hours
    b. 15 hours
    c. 20 hours
    d. 25 hours
    e. There is no CPE requirement

80. What is the maximum amount of pseudoephedrine that can be sold over the counter to an individual on a given day?
    a. 2 grams
    b. 3.2 grams
    c. 3.6 grams
    d. 5 grams
    e. 8 grams

81. What is the maximum amount of pseudoephedrine that can be sold over the counter to an individual over a 30-day period?
    a. 3.6 grams
    b. 5 grams
    c. 8 grams
    d. 8.6 grams
    e. 9 grams

82. A prescription for pseudoephedrine 30mg #120 tablets was dispensed by the pharmacy. The prescription for pseudoephedrine:
    a. Does not need to be reported
    b. Must be reported to NPLEx
    c. Must be reported to the commission
    d. Must be reported to the DEA
    e. Must be reported to the Board of Pharmacy

83. Which DEA form is required for a pharmacy to fill out when ordering Schedule II controlled substances?
    a. Form 41
    b. Form 106
    c. Form 222
    d. Form 223
    e. Form 224

84. Which of the following is FALSE regarding the over-the-counter sale of pseudoephedrine?
    a. The purchaser must produce valid government-issued photo identification
    b. The pharmacy must maintain a log of each sale
    c. The pharmacy must record the date and time of purchase
    d. The purchaser must be at least 21 years old
    e. The pharmacy must record the amount and description of product sold

85. Which of the following statements is/are true regarding syringe and needle sales?

    I. A prescription is required to purchase syringes and needles

    II. Syringe and needle sales are restricted to the pharmacy

    III. An individual may purchase syringes and needles without having a prescription

    a. I only
    b. II only
    c. III only
    d. I and II only
    e. II and III only

86. Which of the following options is/are acceptable for a nuclear pharmacist to certify their training? Select ALL that apply.
    a. Certification of at least 6 months of on-the-job training
    b. Completion of a nuclear pharmacy training program from an accredited college of pharmacy
    c. Completion of a nuclear pharmacy training program from an unaccredited college of pharmacy, with approval from the board
    d. Certification of at least 1 month of training at a nuclear pharmacy
    e. No certification is required to become a nuclear pharmacist

87. In an emergency situation where a Schedule II controlled substance is dispensed by verbal order but there is insufficient stock, how soon shall the rest of the partial fill be dispensed?
    a. Within 24 hours
    b. Within 36 hours
    c. Within 48 hours
    d. Within 72 hours
    e. The partial fill is not permitted and a new prescription would be required

88. Which of the following entities is/are required to be licensed as a wholesaler in Washington state? Select ALL that apply.
    a. In-state pharmaceutical wholesalers
    b. Out-of-state manufacturers that distribute or sell drugs into Washington state
    c. Virtual wholesalers
    d. Reverse distributors
    e. Outsourcing facilities that are required to be registered with the FDA as an outsourcing facility and located in Washington

89. A patient is requesting a refill on a non-controlled prescription that has run out of refills. The pharmacist has attempted but is unable to reach the prescriber. The pharmacist is permitted to renew the non-controlled prescription once within what time period?
    a. 24 months
    b. 12 months
    c. 6 months
    d. 3 months
    e. The pharmacist is not permitted to renew this prescription

90. Which of the following is/are true of drug substitution in an institutional facility?

   I.   Drug substitution is permitted as long as the prescriber is licensed in the state

   II. Drug substitution is permitted without consultation if there is a formulary developed by an interdisciplinary team

   III. The drug formulary listing permitted substitutions is readily retrievable by the pharmacist

   a. I only
   b. II only
   c. III only
   d. II and III only
   e. I, II, and III

91. Which of the following statements is/are true regarding after-hours delivery?

   I.   After-hours delivery is not permitted under any circumstances

   II. Filled prescriptions may be picked up for delivery by authorized personnel when the pharmacy is closed

   III. Prescriptions for after-hours delivery must be placed in a secured delivery area

   a. I only
   b. II only
   c. III only
   d. II and III only
   e. I, II, and III

92. Which of the following professions has unrestricted prescribing authority?
   a. Naturopathic doctor
   b. Physician
   c. Optometrist
   d. Veterinarian
   e. Certified registered nurse anesthetist

93. Which of the following prescriptions needs to be submitted to the prescription monitoring program (PMP)?
    a. A controlled substance provided through inpatient services at a hospital
    b. A controlled substance dispensed at a correctional institution's pharmacy
    c. A controlled substance prescribed for less than a 24-hour supply
    d. A controlled substance prescribed for a 30-day supply
    e. A controlled substance given as a single dose at a hospital's outpatient surgery center

94. What condition(s) must be met when storing drugs in designated areas outside the pharmacy? Select ALL that apply.
    a. Drugs stored in designated areas must be routinely monitored by the supplying pharmacy
    b. Access must be limited to approved health care professionals
    c. Perpetual inventory of all drugs must be kept in the designated drug area
    d. The area must be equipped to ensure security and protection from diversion or tampering
    e. The supplying pharmacy must develop and implement policies and procedures for storing drugs outside the pharmacy

95. If a Schedule II controlled substance is verbally ordered in an emergency, the practitioner must deliver a signed prescription to the dispenser within how many days?
    a. 3 days
    b. 5 days
    c. 7 days
    d. 10 days
    e. 14 days

96. All of the following are examples of prescription adaptation EXCEPT:
    a. Pharmacist changes the quantity if the package size is not commercially available
    b. Pharmacist changes the quantity to coordinate a patient's medication synchronization program
    c. Pharmacist changes the dosage form
    d. Pharmacist completes missing information when there is evidence to support the change
    e. Pharmacist changes the date written

97. How soon do pharmacies need to submit controlled substance dispensing data to the prescription monitoring program (PMP)?
    a. Not later than 1 business day
    b. Not later than 3 business days
    c. Within 24 hours
    d. Within 48 hours
    e. Within 7 days

98. Health care providers with prescriptive authority may prescribe epinephrine to which of the following authorized entities? Select ALL that apply.
    a. Restaurant
    b. Amusement park
    c. Sports arena
    d. Recreation camp
    e. University

99. All of the following may prescribe buprenorphine for opioid dependency treatment EXCEPT:
    a. Physician (MD)
    b. Physician (DO)
    c. Nurse practitioner (NP), through a waiver
    d. Physician assistant (PA), through a waiver
    e. Pharmacist (PharmD), through a waiver

100. A pharmacist in Washington may dispense which of the following prescriptions? Select ALL that apply.
    a. A controlled substance prescription written by an MD in Montana
    b. A non-controlled prescription written by an advanced registered nurse practitioner in California
    c. A controlled substance prescription written by an Optometrist in Oregon
    d. A non-controlled prescription written by a physician assistant in British Columbia
    e. A controlled substance prescription written by an MD in British Columbia

Answer Index – Federal Questions

1 – a

The Food, Drug, and Cosmetic Act (FDCA) requires all new drugs to be proven safe for their labeled use before they can be marketed to patients. This act was passed in 1938 after a drug called elixir sulfanilamide caused mass poisonings and over a hundred deaths in the United States.

2 – a

Drug recalls are classified as Class I, II, or III, from most severe to least severe. A Class I recall is when a product may cause serious adverse health issues or death. A Class II recall is when a product has a low likelihood of causing serious adverse effects, but may cause some temporary or reversible adverse effects. A Class III recall is when a product is not likely to cause adverse health consequences.

3 – d

The Drug Enforcement Administration (DEA) is part of the U.S. Department of Justice and is responsible for the federal CSA. The Controlled Substances Act is available online on the DEA website. HIPAA is usually enforced by the Department of Health and Human Services.

4 – d

The Orange Book (the official title is "Approved Drug Products with Therapeutic Equivalence Evaluations") is the primary source for determining the therapeutic equivalency of drugs. The Purple Book lists biological products that are considered biosimilars and provides interchangeability evaluations for these products. The Red Book contains drug pricing information. The Green Book is for FDA-approved animal drugs.

5 – d

No directions for administration are necessary for oral drug products. However, if drugs are not for oral use, then the specific route(s) of administration must be stated.

Label requirements for the manufacturer container include: name and address of the manufacturer/packer/distributor, name of drug or product, net quantity packaged, weights of each active ingredient, route(s) of administration for non-oral medications, manufacturer control or lot number, expiration date, special storage instructions if applicable, and the federal legend (e.g. "Rx only").

6 – b

According to the DEA Pharmacist's Manual, a controlled substance listed in schedules II, III, IV, or V which is not a prescription drug as determined under the Federal Food, Drug, and Cosmetic Act may be dispensed by a pharmacist to a purchaser at retail, provided that:

- The dispensing is made only by a pharmacist and not by a non–pharmacist employee even if under the supervision of a pharmacist (although after the pharmacist has fulfilled his or her professional and legal responsibilities, the actual cash transaction, credit transaction, or delivery may be completed by a non-pharmacist)

- Not more than 240 cc. (8 ounces) of any such controlled substance containing opium, nor more than 120 cc. (4 ounces) of any other such controlled substance, nor more than 48 dosage units of any such controlled substance containing opium, nor more than 24 dosage units of any other such controlled substance, may be dispensed at retail to the same purchaser in any given 48-hour period

- The purchaser is at least 18 years of age

- The pharmacist requires every purchaser of a controlled substance not known to him to furnish suitable identification (including proof of age where appropriate)

- A bound record book is maintained by the pharmacist which contains the name and address of the purchaser, the name and quantity of the controlled substance purchased, the date of each purchase, and the name or initials of the pharmacist who dispensed the substance to the purchaser

- A prescription is not required for distribution or dispensing of the substance pursuant to any other federal, state or local law

- Central fill pharmacies may not dispense controlled substances at the retail level to a purchaser.

7 – a

A DEA Form 106, titled "Report of Theft or Loss of Controlled Substances," is a form that must be filled out and submitted to the DEA upon discovery of theft or significant loss of controlled substances. There is a section of the DEA Form 106 that allows the user to list out the controlled substances and quantities that were stolen or lost. Submitting a DEA Form 106 formally documents the situation and the pharmacy should retain a copy for their records. The DEA must also immediately be contacted by phone, fax, or brief written message to alert them of the situation. The local authorities should also be alerted.

There is no DEA Form 108. DEA Form 222 is for ordering Schedule II controlled substances. DEA Form 224 is for registration with the DEA. DEA Form 363 is for narcotic treatment facilities.

8 – d

Pentobarbital is a Schedule II controlled substance. It is a barbiturate. Schedule II controlled substances include but are not limited to: opiates and opioids, amphetamines and dextroamphetamine salts, pentobarbital, secobarbital, and phencyclidine. Mescaline is a Schedule I controlled substance. Butabarbital is a Schedule III controlled substance. Modafinil is a Schedule IV controlled substance. Finally, buprenorphine is a Schedule III controlled substance.

9 – c

A water-containing oral formulation made from commercially available drug products has a maximum BUD of 14 days when stored in the refrigerator. Non-aqueous formulations have a maximum BUD of 6 months. Water-containing topical/dermals, mucosal liquids, and semisolid formulations have a maximum beyond-use-date of 30 days.

Drugs or chemicals that are known to be labile to decomposition will require shorter BUDs. Finally, the BUD cannot exceed the expiration date of the active pharmaceutical ingredient (API) or any other component in the product.

10 – c

Here is a summary of DEA forms to know:

- DEA Form 222 is for ordering Schedule I or II controlled substances

- DEA Form 224 is for registering a new pharmacy

- DEA Form 363 is for new registration applications for narcotic treatment programs

- DEA Form 106 is for reporting loss

- DEA Form 41 is for drug destruction.

11 – c

The Food and Drug Administration has developed four distinct approaches to making certain types of new drugs available as rapidly as possible. The four approaches are:

- Fast track

- Breakthrough therapy

- Accelerated approval

- Priority review

Fast track is an expedited review process intended for drugs that treat serious conditions and fill an unmet medical need. Breakthrough therapy is a process designed to expedite the development and review of drugs which may demonstrate substantial improvement over available therapy. Accelerated approval is for drugs with long-term endpoints that are hard to measure during clinical trials, such as a decrease in mortality or increase in survival. These drugs are approved based on a surrogate endpoint. Finally, the priority review designation means the FDA's goal is to take action on the application within six months. "Instant approval" is not an FDA process.

12 - d

Schedule II controlled substances can be transferred in all of the given scenarios except for a researcher transferring Schedule II controlled substances to a pharmacy to be dispensed to patients. Researchers must be authorized to conduct research with Schedule II controlled substances. Researchers may transfer Schedule II controlled substances to another authorized researcher for the purpose of research. Researchers may not transfer Schedule II controlled substances to a pharmacy.

13 – b

Once a pharmacy has filled and dispensed a medication, the prescription is legally owned by the pharmacy and the original prescription can't be returned to the patient. However, it is acceptable to make a copy for the patient or the prescriber if needed. The prescription can be transferred to another pharmacy (if legal depending on the schedule and number of refills remaining), but the pharmacy that originally filled the prescription must retain the original copy.

14 - b

When purchasing Schedule II controlled substances, the pharmacy (purchaser) will fill out a DEA Form 222 and submit it to the supplier. The supplier receives the original form. The purchaser is required to make a copy of the original DEA Form 222 for their records. This copy can be retained in paper or electronic form. The purchaser does not have the option of keeping the original form.

15 – b

A Class II drug recall occurs when the product may cause temporary or medically reversible adverse effects, but the probability of serious adverse effects is remote.

16 – c

National Drug Codes (NDCs) are drug identification numbers that are unique to each drug manufactured. The NDC contains 3 sets of numbers:

1) The first set is either a 4- or 5-digit number and represents the manufacturer.

2) The second set is a 4-digit number that represents the identity of the drug.

3) The third set is a 2-digit number that is the product package size, such as the bottle count, blister packs, etc.

For example, we might have levothyroxine 50 mcg that is supplied as a 100-count bottle and a 500-count bottle from the same manufacturer. The NDC code will be the same except for the last 2 numbers because the bottle count sizes are different.

17 – e

Good Manufacturing Practice (GMP) is a set of regulations that determines minimum standards for pharmaceutical manufacturing in the U.S. The purpose of GMP is to uphold the safety and quality of drug products.

18 – b

According to the DEA Pharmacist's Manual, these are the criteria for an individual practitioner issuing multiple prescriptions for up to a 90-day supply of a Schedule II controlled substance:

- Each separate prescription is issued for a legitimate medical purpose by an individual practitioner acting in the usual course of professional practice

- The individual practitioner provides written instructions on each prescription (other than the first prescription, if the prescribing practitioner intends for that prescription to be filled immediately) indicating the earliest <u>date</u> on which a pharmacy may fill each prescription

- The individual practitioner concludes that providing the patient with multiple prescriptions in this manner does not create an undue risk of diversion or abuse

- The issuance of multiple prescriptions is permissible under the applicable state laws

- The individual practitioner complies fully with all other applicable federal requirements as well as any additional requirements under state law.

19 – d

Based on federal law, Schedule III and IV controlled substances can be filled up to 5 times in a 6-month period from the date the prescription was written. Some states also apply this refill rule to Schedule V controlled substances. When a refill is dispensed for a Schedule III or IV substance, the dispensing pharmacist's initials, date the prescription was refilled, and amount of drug dispensed must be documented. Review page 49 of the 2022 version of the DEA Pharmacist's manual for information about the electronic recordkeeping of Schedules III–IV refill information.

20 – d

Section 1262 of the Consolidated Appropriations Act of 2023 removes the federal requirement for practitioners to apply for a special waiver ("X" number) prior to prescribing buprenorphine for the treatment of opioid use disorder.

21 – b

Adulteration involves the integrity and composition of a product. If the composition or integrity of a drug is compromised, then the drug is considered adulterated. Some examples of adulteration include:

- A drug contains a decomposed substance

- A drug that is not manufactured under required manufacturing standards

- A drug that is stored in unsanitary conditions

- A substance of the drug container leaches into the drug itself

- A drug that is not pure or contains less than the listed amount of active ingredient

- A drug that contains an unapproved color additive.

22 – d

According to the Code of Federal Regulations, mid-level practitioners are defined as individual practitioners other than physicians, dentists, veterinarians, or podiatrists. Mid-level practitioners include but are not limited to: nurse practitioners, nurse midwives, nurse anesthetists, clinical nurse specialists, physician assistants, optometrists, homeopathic physicians, registered pharmacists, and certified chiropractors.

23 – a, d, e

DME is made for long-term use and must be able to withstand repeated use, be primarily for a medical purpose, and be appropriate for home use. It includes many different types of devices for individuals with a variety of conditions. Some examples of durable medical equipment include wheelchairs, crutches, canes, oxygen, ventilators, and hospital beds.

24 – a

The Prescription Drug Marketing Act (PDMA) of 1987 involves several laws regarding prescription drugs. Primarily, it regulates the storage, distribution, and resale of drug samples. It enforces recordkeeping requirements for prescription drug samples. The PDMA also prohibits hospitals and other health care entities from reselling their drugs to other businesses. This is because hospitals usually obtain drugs at a special rate. Finally, it regulates state licensing of wholesalers.

25 – a, b, c

An NDC number is a numeric, 3-segment code that identifies a drug by manufacturer (first 4 or 5 numbers), specific drug (next 4 numbers), and package (last 2 numbers). NDC numbers are unique to each drug and serve as a universal product identifier for drugs. The expiration date information is not included in the NDC number. By law, the FDA does not require that drug manufacturers include NDC numbers on labels, but it is highly recommended.

NDC numbers are published in an NDC Directory by the FDA. The labeler is responsible for the content of the NDC entry, not the FDA. Therefore, inclusion of information in the NDC directory doesn't mean that the FDA has verified the information. Additionally, assignment of an NDC number does not mean the drug has been approved by the FDA.

26 – a

Isotretinoin is an oral medication used to treat severe acne. Taking isotretinoin during pregnancy can cause birth defects, therefore this drug is highly regulated through a REMS program.

The REMS program for isotretinoin is called iPLEDGE. Under iPLEDGE:

- Only doctors registered with iPLEDGE may prescribe isotretinoin

- Only patients registered with iPLEDGE may receive isotretinoin

- Only pharmacies registered with iPLEDGE may dispense isotretinoin

- Patients may receive no more than a 30-day supply at a time

- No refills are allowed on prescriptions for isotretinoin

- Female patients who can get pregnant must use 2 separate methods of effective birth control 1 month before, while taking, and for 1 month after taking isotretinoin

- Female patients who can get pregnant must take a pregnancy test every month.

27 – b

Compounded drugs cannot be compounded, provided, or sold to other pharmacies or third parties. Compounded drugs cannot be commercially available, must meet national standards, must be a reasonable quantity for current or anticipated prescriptions, and distribution cannot be more than 5% of total prescriptions filled by the pharmacy per year. Drugs that have been removed from the market cannot be used in compounding.

Compounding may be an option to customize medications based upon a doctor's prescription. For example, compounding can customize a drug strength, remove an allergenic component, flavor a medication, and change the dosage form.

28 – b

A DEA Form 222 or an electronically equivalent program is necessary in order to purchase or transfer Schedule II controlled substances.

29 – d

The Schedule II controlled substance prescription can be mailed to the patient. Controlled substances used to not be able to be mailed, but this is no longer the case. The package must contain an inner package with the prescription and appropriate labeling, but must be placed in a plain outer container. The outside package cannot contain information about the contents of the package.

30 – c

Narrow therapeutic index drugs are drugs where small differences in the dose or blood concentration may lead to serious therapeutic failures or adverse reactions. These drugs require careful titration or patient monitoring for safe and effective use. They are permitted to be prescribed.

Some drugs with a narrow therapeutic index are: warfarin, levothyroxine, digoxin, lithium carbonate, phenytoin, and cyclosporine. Additionally, the FDA recommends that potency of the drug have a variability limit of 90% to 105% when the drugs are manufactured.

31 – a

The Poison Prevention Packaging Act (PPPA) set the requirement that prescription drugs, non-prescription drugs, and hazardous household products must have a child-resistant closure. The purpose was to protect children less than 5 years old from poisoning from accidental ingestion or exposure.

Patients may ask to not have safety caps on their medications, especially if they have conditions such as arthritis that make it difficult for them to open up the containers.

There are also several prescription drugs that are exempt from PPPA, such as nitroglycerin sublingual tablets, oral contraceptives in mnemonic dispenser packages, isosorbide dinitrate in sublingual and chewable forms, and more.

32 – a

The Combat Methamphetamine Epidemic Act of 2005 is a federal law that regulates "regulated sellers" including most pharmacies. It sets forth the requirements that these sellers must follow in order to sell ephedrine, pseudoephedrine, and phenylpropanolamine over the counter. Here are some requirements to know:

1) Products must be placed behind the counter or in locked cabinets

2) The identity of the purchasers must be verified, and a log of each sale must be obtained

3) The log must contain:
   - Purchaser's name
   - Address
   - Signature of the purchaser
   - Product sold
   - Quantity sold
   - Date
   - Time

4) The logbook must be kept for 2 years

5) All employees must be trained in the requirements and certify that they have received training

6) The quantity limits are 3.6 grams per day and 9 grams in a 30-day period. No more than 7.5 grams can be imported by mail

7) The logbook requirement does not apply to individual single sales packages of no more than 60 milligrams of pseudoephedrine

The DEA Pharmacist's Manual gives a complete list of proof-of-identity requirements.

33 – a

OTC drug advertising is regulated by the Federal Trade Commission (FTC). Prescription drug advertising is regulated by the Food and Drug Administration (FDA).

34 – c

Under the Drug Supply Chain Security Act, manufacturers are required to provide a transaction report (pedigree) for each product sold. Pharmacies are required to receive this information and pass it along if they further distribute the product. This allows the drugs to be tracked. The transaction report includes 3 parts, also known informally as the "3 T's": transaction information, transaction history, and transaction statement.

35 – e

The Kefauver-Harris Amendment requires that manufacturers provide proof of the effectiveness and safety of their drugs before these drugs can be approved. This was the first "proof-of-efficacy" requirement. The situation that prompted this amendment was the use of thalidomide in Europe that was marketed as a sedative-hypnotic drug that could be used during pregnancy, but it caused serious birth defects. Before the Kefauver-Harris Amendment, the Food, Drug, and Cosmetic Act (FDCA) of 1939 required drugs to be proven safe before being marketed.

36 – c

Pharmacies will use DEA Form 224 to register with the DEA to possess and dispense controlled substances. DEA Form 106 is to report theft or loss of controlled substances. DEA Form 222 to order and transfer Schedule I and II controlled substances. DEA Form 225 is used by manufacturers, distributors, importers, exporters, and researchers to register to conduct business with controlled substances. DEA Form 363 is used by narcotic treatment programs to register to conduct business with controlled substances.

37 – b

A drug product that is manufactured in the U.S., then exported to a foreign country, and then re-imported back to the U.S., is only legal if it is done by the original manufacturer. Re-importation is permitted by the original manufacturer if the purpose is for emergency medical care. Otherwise, re-importation of drugs is not permitted.

Some consumers want to engage in drug re-importation because drugs may be sold at a lower price outside of the United States. It would be a way to obtain access to these lower drug prices from countries such as Canada and Mexico, but it is illegal.

38 – b

Methadone is used for both the treatment of pain (i.e., as an analgesic) and in the detoxification and maintenance of narcotic addiction in patients registered in a narcotic treatment program. While a retail pharmacy may stock methadone, methadone can only be dispensed as an analgesic. Methadone can only be dispensed for the maintenance or detoxification of addicts when it is provided through a registered narcotic treatment center. It can be provided through one of these centers for either short-term detoxification (up to 30 days) or long-term detoxification (30–180 days).

39 – c

The Safe Medical Device Act (SMDA) of 1990 requires health care facilities to report death or injuries caused by or suspected to have been caused by a medical device to the FDA or the manufacturer. The goal is to quickly inform the FDA on the issue so the product can be tracked and potentially recalled for safety reasons. Some examples of medical devices that could be reported are: defibrillators, shunts, lab reagents, pulse oximeters, glucose meters, infusion pumps, wheelchairs, ventilator breathing circuits, needles, and catheters.

40 – c

Misbranding is inaccurate labeling on the drug container. If information is missing, inaccurate, or untrue, this is considered misbranding.

Examples of misbranding include: false or misleading information, unreadable material, omitting a medication guide, inadequate directions or warnings, omitting required information, etc.

41 – a, b, c

According to the Controlled Substances Act, a prescription for a controlled substance must:

1) Be dated and signed on the issue date

2) Include:
   - Patient's full name and address
   - Practitioner's full name, address and DEA number
   - Drug name
   - Drug strength
   - Dosage form
   - Quantity prescribed
   - Directions for use
   - Number of refills authorized
   - Manual signature of the practitioner

3) Be issued for a legitimate medical purpose by a practitioner acting in the usual course of professional practice

4) Not be issued in order for an individual practitioner to obtain a supply of controlled substances to keep on hand for the purpose of general dispensing to patients

Note: Even though the prescriber is responsible for ensuring that the controlled substance prescription is up to the lawful standard, a corresponding responsibility rests with the pharmacist who fills the prescription.

42 – c

A drug (or biologic) is considered to be an orphan drug if it is intended to treat a rare disease or condition that impacts fewer than 200,000 people in the U.S.

Sometimes, an orphan drug designation can be given to drugs citing a cost recovery provision, which is if the cost of research and development of the drug is not reasonably expected to be regained by sales of the drug.

43 – b

Several ingredients such as FD&C Yellow No. 5, aspartame, wintergreen oil, mineral oil, salicylates, sulfites, Ipecac syrup, and alcohol have special labeling requirements under federal regulations. FD&C Yellow No. 5, also called tartrazine, is a color additive that may cause an allergic reaction (itching and hives) in some people. Therefore, a product that contains FD&C Yellow No. 5 must identify so on the label.

44 – e

Normally, a faxed prescription for a Schedule II controlled substance cannot be accepted. However, there are 3 exceptions. Prescriptions for Schedule II controlled substances can be faxed and serve as the original prescription for patients residing in a long-term care facility, enrolled in hospice, or if the drug is to be compounded for direct administration by parenteral, intravenous, intramuscular, subcutaneous, or intraspinal infusion (which includes home infusion therapy).

45 – b

The FDA Adverse Event Reporting System (FAERS) is a database where adverse events from medications can be voluntarily reported. This provides post-marketing safety surveillance on medications.

Meanwhile, the VAERS stands for the Vaccine Adverse Event Reporting System, which is a national vaccine safety surveillance program run by the CDC and FDA.

ERSA, MAERS, and AERS are not drug-related reporting systems.

46 – c

A prescription for a Schedule II controlled substance can be called in orally to be dispensed in an emergency situation. The prescription should be immediately written down by the pharmacist. The quantity should only be enough to adequately cover the emergency period. The pharmacy needs to receive a hard copy prescription from the prescriber within 7 days after authorizing the emergency dispensing. This must also have the words "authorization for emergency dispensing" on the prescription and the date of the oral order written on the front. Prescriptions postmarked within the 7-day period are acceptable. If the prescription is not received in a timely manner, this should be reported to the DEA.

47 – b

The Purple Book contains information related to biological products and information regarding interchangeable biological products. The Orange Book provides information regarding therapeutic equivalence between drugs (excluding biologics). The Red Book is used for drug pricing and packaging information. The Pink Book contains information related to immunizations and vaccine-preventable diseases, as well as information on vaccine safety. Information and recommendation related to international travel (vaccines, diseases, information of other health risks) can be bound in the Yellow Book.

48 – e

An exact count must be made on controlled substances if they are Schedule I or II controlled substances, if they are controlled substances where the bottles contain more than 1000 tablets or capsules, and if the containers are sealed or unopened. Sealed or unopened containers do not need to be opened and counted, but the number marked as the container quantity must be used as an exact count.

49 – b

The U.S. Attorney General, as head of the Justice Department (which the Drug Enforcement Administration is under), may add, delete, or reschedule substances. A scientific and medical recommendation from the Food and Drug Administration is included in the decision.

50 – c

A full NDA must be submitted to the FDA when a manufacturer wants to request reclassification of a current prescription-only drug to be an over-the-counter drug. This is just one method of requesting reclassification, as there are four different methods. Another method is the FDA granting an exemption if determining prescription-only status is not necessary for the safety and protection of the public. A third method is filing a supplement to the original NDA (a "supplemental NDA") for review of the drug's safety and adverse events. The last method is if the Nonprescription Drug Advisory Committee recommends the ingredient contained in the drug be converted to a non-prescription status.

An ANDA is an application for the potential approval of a generic drug product. Both EIND and IND are applications regarding the development of a new drug. A marketed new drug application is not an existing type of application.

51 – a

In order to verify a DEA number, use the following process:

1) Add together the first, third, and fifth numbers.

2) Add together the second, fourth, and sixth numbers. Multiply this number by two.

3) Add the numbers together from steps 1 and 2. The last digit of the number you get from step 3 is the last number of the DEA number.

Using the DEA number BS5927683, the process would be:

1) $5 + 2 + 6 = 13$

2) $(9 + 7 + 8) \times 2 = (24) \times 2 = 48$

3) $13 + 48 = 61 \rightarrow$ Since the last digit is 1, the DEA should end in 1, not 3.

52 – d

Dentists must prescribe within their scope of practice. Accordingly, prescriptions written by a dentist must treat a disease of the mouth, treat discomfort of the mouth, or be used to facilitate a dental procedure. Atorvastatin is used to lower cholesterol. Other professions, such as optometrists and veterinarians, must also prescribe within their scope of practice.

53 – e

A DEA Form 222 must be signed and dated by the person authorized to sign the pharmacy's DEA registration. This means that only the pharmacist who signed the most recent application for renewal of the pharmacy's DEA registration may sign a DEA Form 222. Additionally, that pharmacist may authorize others to sign a DEA Form 222 by granting a power of attorney. A power of attorney must be signed by the registrant (the person granting the power), the person to whom the power of attorney is being granted, and two witnesses.

54 – b

Phase 1 clinical trials are conducted in a small group of healthy participants without the disease condition. Typically, the study size is around 20–80 people. The goal of the Phase 1 clinical trial is to study the properties of the drug and determine safety. Sometimes the Phase 1 clinical trial can include participants with the disease condition, but this is not as common.

Phase 2 clinical trials are conducted in a larger size group of 100 or more people, and these participants have the disease condition. Phase 2 clinical trials study the effectiveness of the drug.

Phase 3 clinical trials are conducted in a larger group of hundreds or thousands of participants who have the disease condition. The drug's safety, efficacy, and dosing are further studied. If a drug passes the Phase 3 study, then it can be approved by the FDA.

Finally, Phase 4 clinical trials are conducted after the drug is approved and looks at the safety and efficacy of the drug long-term, also called post-marketing surveillance.

55 – c

A pharmacy may keep shipping and financial data for controlled substances at a central location other than the registered location after notifying the nearest DEA Diversion Field Office. Executed DEA Form 222 orders, controlled substance prescriptions, and controlled substance inventories must be kept at the pharmacy location that is registered with the DEA and cannot be kept at a central location.

56 – c

Schedule III controlled substances have less potential for abuse than Schedule I or II drugs, and they have a currently accepted medical use in the U.S. Codeine by itself is classified under Schedule II, but in combination with acetaminophen it is a Schedule III drug.

57 – e

HIPAA permits the use of protected health information (PHI) for treatment purposes. Medical information can be shared to persons involved in the patient's care without written or verbal consent.

58 – b

The Federal Transfer Warning ("Caution: Federal law prohibits the transfer of this drug to any person other than the patient for whom it was prescribed") is required on the label of Schedule II–IV controlled substances when dispensed to a patient. Most pharmacies comply with this requirement by including this warning on all prescription labels. However, it is not legally required on prescription labels for Schedule V controlled substances and non-controlled prescriptions.

59 – a

Outsourcing facilities, also known as 503B facilities, are permitted to compound sterile products without receiving patient-specific prescriptions or medication orders. They are regulated by the FDA and subject to current good manufacturing practices. Compounded products must be distributed within a health care setting or dispensed directly to a patient or prescriber, and may not be sold or transferred to a wholesaler for redistribution.

A pharmacy that registers as an outsourcing facility would therefore be able to compound sterile products without receiving patient-specific prescriptions.

60 – b, c, e

The Health Information Technology for Economic and Clinical Health Act (HITECH Act) promotes health information technology to advance healthcare and the use of electronic health records. The HIPAA Breach Notification Rule is a part of this act.

It requires entities to notify affected individuals without unreasonable delay, and in no case later than 60 days following the discovery of a breach of unsecured protected health information. Breaches of 500 or more records also need to be reported to the Secretary of the U.S. Department of Health and Human Services (HHS) within 60 days of the discovery of the breach, and smaller breaches within 60 days of the end of the calendar year in which the breach occurred. In addition to reporting the breach to the HHS Secretary, a notice of a breach of 500 or more records must be provided to prominent media outlets serving the state or jurisdiction affected by the breach.

61 – d

The USP Chapter <797> describes the requirements of sterile compounded preparations, including responsibilities of compounding personnel, training, facilities, environmental monitoring, and storage and testing. USP Chapter <795> covers nonsterile compounding, and USP Chapter <800> describes safe handling of hazardous drugs. USP <503A> and USP <503B> do not exist as USP chapters; however, the terms 503A and 503B are used to designate compounding pharmacies.

62 – b, c, d

Every person or firm that manufactures, distributes, or dispenses any controlled substance must register with the DEA. However, patients who receive controlled substance prescriptions and pharmacists working in a pharmacy are exempt from DEA registration requirements. Therefore, pharmacists do not need to have a DEA number to dispense controlled substances.

63 – b

Clozapine is associated with severe neutropenia, which can lead to severe infections. Prescribers are required to be certified in the clozapine REMS program before prescribing clozapine. Pharmacies are also required to be certified in the clozapine REMS program to dispense clozapine.

64 – c

A DEA Form 41 is used to document the destruction of controlled substances. More commonly, a pharmacy will transfer controlled substances to an authorized reverse distributor for destruction. The reverse distributor then fills out DEA Form 41 to document the destruction of controlled substances.

65 – b

The Federal Anti-Tampering Act requires tamper-evident packaging of many over-the-counter products and cosmetics to avoid contamination issues and limit access. If the items were tampered with, it would be evident due to the packaging of these products. For example, some products have a tamper-evident closure cap, tamper-evident liner, and tamper-evident tape. The act was passed in response to the Tylenol poisoning deaths in Chicago in 1982, where the Tylenol capsules were contaminated with cyanide.

66 – a

Schedule I controlled substances include drugs that have a high potential for abuse and severe potential for dependence, with no currently accepted medical use in the U.S. This includes heroin, lysergic acid diethylamide (LSD), mescaline, and methaqualone, among others.

67 – c

Manufacturer's containers of OTC medications are required to display the following information: identity of the product (active ingredient), inactive ingredient(s), purpose, use(s), warnings, directions, and storage information.

Other information that is not required, but may be included, is as follows: net quantity of contents, name and address of the manufacturer/packager/distributor, lot number or batch code, expiration date, and instructions for what to do if an overdose occurs.

While the Poison Control Center phone number is included on some OTC medications, it is not required by federal law.

68 – b

Patient Package Inserts (PPIs) must be provided to patients in acute-care hospitals or long-term care facilities prior to the first administration and every 30 days thereafter. They are required for oral contraceptives and estrogen-containing products.

69 – c

DEA registration permits pharmacies, manufacturers, distributors, importers, exporters, and researchers to possess controlled substances. A DEA registration is valid for 36 months. Registrants will receive renewal notification approximately 60 days prior to the DEA registration expiration date.

70 – c

For recordkeeping requirements, executed copies of DEA Form 222 must be maintained separately from all other records. If a pharmacy stores these forms electronically, then the electronic records are deemed separate if such copies are readily retrievable from all other electronic records. A defective DEA Form 222 cannot be corrected and needs to be replaced by a new form. Finally, when filling out the DEA Form 222, only 1 item may be entered on each numbered line.

71 – e

Under the Health Insurance Portability and Accountability Act (HIPAA) Privacy Rule, a communication is not considered "marketing" if it is made for the treatment of the individual. Therefore, refill reminders for currently prescribed medications (or one that has not lapsed for more than 90 days) are not considered marketing. Therefore, offering this service is not a HIPAA violation. Patients may be charged for this service as long as any payment made to the pharmacy is reasonable and related to the pharmacy's cost of making the communication. Mailed refill reminders are valid, as well as electronic refill reminders.

As a note, the HIPAA Privacy Rule defines marketing as making "a communication about a product or service that encourages recipients of the communication to purchase or use the product or service." An entity would need to receive authorization from the patient to send out marketing communications.

72 – d

Manufacturer's expiration dates may be expressed as a day, month, and year, or as just a month and year. If it is written as only month and year, the drug expires on the last day of the listed month. The drug is safe to use on the expiration date, but not after.

73 – c

A prospective DUR consists of reviewing a prescription for adverse effects, therapeutic duplication, drug-disease interactions and contraindications, drug dosing and regimen, drug allergies, clinical misuse or abuse, drug interactions, medication appropriateness, overutilization, underutilization, and pregnancy alerts. Ensuring compliance with prescription labeling is not part of the prospective DUR.

74 – a

The purpose of the Federal Hazardous Substances Act (FHSA) is to protect consumers from hazardous or toxic substances. The FHSA requires precautionary labeling on the immediate container of hazardous household products, which includes certain OTC medications. Medication packages would include the statement, "Keep out of the reach of children." Depending on the hazardous substance, additional warnings and statements, such as "handle with gloves" or "harmful if swallowed," may be required. The warning "Keep out of the reach of children" applies to OTC drugs and not FDA-regulated drugs.

75 – c

The 5% rule states that a pharmacy does not have to register with the DEA as a distributor if the total quantity of controlled substances distributed during a 12-month period does not exceed 5% of the total quantity of all controlled substances dispensed and distributed during that period.

76 – d

The Occupational and Safety Health Administration (OSHA) requires that employers meet the Hazardous Communication Standard. This includes having a Hazardous Communication Plan, which lists hazardous chemicals in the workplace, and ensuring that all such products are appropriately labeled and have a Safety Data Sheet. Workers must be trained on the hazards of chemicals, appropriate protective measures, and where to find more information. The purpose of OSHA is to protect employees, which is separate from laws intended to protect consumers and patients.

77 – b

The Consumer Product Safety Commission administers the Poison Prevention Packaging Act (PPPA). This act requires child-resistant containers for all prescriptions and certain non-prescription drugs, unless there is an exemption for a specific drug or circumstance.

78 – d

Bulk compounding of products in order to sell them to other pharmacies is considered "manufacturing," which is regulated by the FDA. Note that for manufacturing, a patient-specific prescription is not required. So, in this case, since there is not a patient-specific prescription involved, the mass production of ibuprofen suppositories is considered manufacturing. On the other hand, "compounding" is typically regulated by state boards of pharmacy and is limited to compounding prescriptions for individual patients pursuant to a prescription.

79 – e

The Prescription Drug Marketing Act bans most pharmacies from purchasing, trading, selling, or possessing prescription drug samples. The only exception is for pharmacies that are owned by a charitable organization or by a city, state, or county government and that are part of a health care entity providing care to indigent or low-income patients at no or reduced cost. In this case, samples may only be provided at no cost to the patients.

80 – e

DEA Form 222 is used to transfer and order Schedule II controlled substances. The DEA used to allow this form to be faxed, but not anymore. A DEA Form 224 is needed for a pharmacy to dispense controlled substances. Schedule III–V controlled substances may be ordered through normal ordering processes from wholesalers or manufacturers, but must be documented by the pharmacy with an invoice upon receipt. The common term used for ordering Schedule III–V controlled substances is "using an invoice."

81 – d

Manufacturers and packagers of over-the-counter drugs for sale at retail must package products in tamper-evident packaging, with some exceptions. The exceptions are dermatological, dentifrice, insulin, or lozenge products.

82 – c

A pharmacist may not change the following items on a Schedule II controlled substance prescription: name of the patient, name of the drug, and name of the prescriber. All other information, including quantity, directions for use, drug strength, and dosage form, may be changed with the verbal permission of the prescriber as long as the change is documented on the prescription.

83 – e

Patients have a right to obtain a copy of their protected health information. Pharmacies must comply with such a request within 30 days. If there is a delay, the patient must be notified of the reason for delay and the pharmacy may extend the time by no more than 30 additional days. Normally, pharmacies are able to give a copy of the prescription record on the day of the request.

84 - b

Thalidomide is an immunomodulatory agent as well as a chemotherapy drug. Thalidomide causes a high frequency of birth defects in pregnant females. Babies were born with missing or deformed arms and legs. Therefore, the REMS program was developed to ensure safe use and monitoring of thalidomide.

85 – c

The Kefauver-Harris Amendment of 1962 is more commonly known as the "Drug Efficacy Amendment." It requires new drugs to be proven as safe and effective before they are approved. It also allows the FDA to establish good drug manufacturing practices and gives the FDA jurisdiction over prescription drug advertising, which must include accurate information about side effects. It also controls the marketing of generic drugs to keep them from being sold as expensive medications under new trade names.

86 – c

Anabolic steroids are classified as Schedule III controlled substances under federal law. An example of an anabolic steroid is testosterone.

87 – d

The Durham-Humphrey Amendment created two separate categories of drugs, prescription (legend) and over-the-counter (OTC). Prescription drugs require a prescription and must be dispensed under medical supervision. OTC drugs can be obtained without a prescription and do not require medical supervision.

88 – d

Generic bioequivalence information is found in the FDA Orange Book. A two-letter coding system indicates equivalency, with the first letter being key. Codes that start with the letter A indicate that the FDA considers the drug products to be pharmaceutically and therapeutically equivalent. Codes that start with the letter B indicate that the FDA does not consider the products to be equivalent.

The second letter of the code typically indicates the dosage form (for example, a code of AT would indicate that two topical products are equivalent).

Products with known or potential equivalency issues, but for which adequate scientific evidence exists to establish bioequivalence, are given a code of AB.

89 – a, b, d

DEA registration is not required for an agent or employee of any registered manufacturer, distributor, or dispenser if acting in the usual course of business. This includes pharmacists working at pharmacies and nurses working in a hospital or physician's office. Patients who possess controlled substances for a lawful purpose are not required to register with the DEA.

Providers must register with the DEA unless practicing under the registration of a hospital or other institution. Each pharmacy must have its own DEA registration to dispense controlled substances.

90 – d

A product is considered adulterated if its strength or quality differs from what it represents (this is not the only criteria for adulteration, but one example). A product is misbranded if the labeling is false or misleading. If a drug product's strength is less than what is represented on the label, then the drug product is considered both adulterated and misbranded.

91 – d

Patients may request easy-open containers (containers that are not child-resistant) for any prescription. A provider may also make this request on a patient's behalf (written or verbal), but can only do so for one individual prescription. Only a patient can issue a blanket request for easy-open containers on all future prescriptions. There is not a legal requirement for documentation of easy-open container requests, but it is good practice for a pharmacist to have documentation in case an issue arises.

92 – c

Risk Evaluation and Mitigation Strategies (REMS) are strategies to manage a known or potential serious risk associated with a drug. A REMS program does not have anything to do with the affordability of drugs.

93 – c

Federal regulations require a warning statement, including a warning about the risk of Reye's syndrome in children, on aspirin and other salicylate products. An example warning statement is: "Keep out of reach of children. In case of overdose, get medical help or contact a Poison Control Center right away." Containers of chewable 81mg (1.25 grain) aspirin may not contain more than 36 tablets in order to reduce the risk of accidental poisoning in children. In other words, if a child were to open a bottle of aspirin and ingest all 36 tablets, 36 tablets would generally be considered a non-toxic amount.

94 – b

DEA registration numbers begin with two letters. The first letter indicates practitioner status, in which "M" is the designation for mid-level practitioners. The second letter typically indicates the first letter of the practitioner's last name, the first letter of the pharmacy name, or the first letter of the hospital name.

To verify the DEA registration number, first add together the 1st, 3rd, and 5th digit. Then add together the 2nd, 4th, and 6th digit, and multiply this number by two. Add these two numbers together. The last digit (in the ones place) of the sum of these two numbers should match the last number of the DEA registration number.

Check each of the five choices. For the second choice (MT1200980):

1) $1 + 0 + 9 = 10$

2) $2 + 0 + 8 = 10$; $10 \times 2 = 20$

3) $10 + 20 = 30$

The last digit of 30 is 0, so 0 must be the last digit of the DEA number: MT1200980.

95 – a, b, d

The FDA requires medication guides be issued with certain prescription drugs and biologics if they determine the drug has serious risks relative to benefits, when patient adherence is crucial to the effectiveness of the drug, when there is a known serious side effect, and when providing information can prevent serious adverse effects. Medication guides do not replace pharmacist counseling. A patient also does not need to be in a nursing home to receive a medication guide. Some drugs which require a guide be dispensed with each fill are: aripiprazole, amphetamine/dextroamphetamine, fentanyl, testosterone, citalopram, ciprofloxacin, amiodarone, duloxetine, adalimumab, and more.

96 – e

Omnibus Budget Reconciliation Act of 1990 (commonly known as OBRA 90) set the requirement that patients must be offered counseling on medications. Patients have the right to refuse this counseling, but counseling must at least be offered.

97 – a, b, e

Several drugs are exempt from the child-resistant container packaging requirement. Some examples include sublingual nitroglycerin tablets, methylprednisolone tablets containing no more than 84mg per package, preparations in aerosol containers intended for inhalation, and more. Effervescent aspirin or acetaminophen tablets are exempt, but non-effervescent tablets are not. Packages of prednisone tablets are only exempt if they contain less than 105mg per package.

98 – b

Prescription records are required to be kept for a minimum of 2 years based on federal law. However, if there are stricter state laws, those should be followed. For example, if a state requires prescription records to be maintained for 5 years, then prescription records must be maintained for at least 5 years because it is stricter than 2 years.

99 – b

Aripiprazole (Abilify) is a drug that has a medication guide. Drugs that pose a serious or significant concern have medication guides. The medication guide is required for each dispensing, including refills. The medication guide is required as part of the labeling. If the medication guide is not given, the drug is considered misbranded.

100 – b

CMS regulations require a consultant pharmacist to perform a drug regimen review for long-term care patients at least once a month.

Answer Index – Washington Questions

1 – a, b

A CDTA is an agreement between a prescriber and a pharmacist. Per WAC 246-945-350, a CDTA allows a pharmacist to prescribe within a certain protocol authorized by a doctor. Prescribed drugs may include legend drugs as well as controlled substances and vaccines.

Pharmacists acting with prescriptive authority to prescribe controlled substances must have their own unique DEA registration number issued by the DEA. The pharmacist may not use the authorizing prescriber's DEA number. There is a variation to this if pharmacists are acting with prescriptive authority in hospitals or other institutional settings.

A CDTA is valid for two years from the date of signing. The commission clarified DEA registration for pharmacists in its April 2018 Newsletter (No. 1283 Practitioner DEA Registrations).

2 – a

Per WAC 246-945-420, when a drug is added to the controlled substance schedule, the pharmacy must conduct an inventory of controlled substances on the effective date that the drug becomes scheduled. The drug then becomes included in the controlled substance inventories thereafter.

3 – c

Per WAC 246-945-445, the director of pharmacy or their designee has responsibility for the distribution of drugs. The pharmacy shall also be responsible for maintaining and providing information on approved investigational drugs. How the investigational drugs are eventually used will depend on the principal investigator or co-investigator(s).

4 – a

Many states have enacted laws pertaining to the schedule and reporting requirements for gabapentin. At this time, Washington has not.

5 - a, c

Per WAC 246-945-425, pharmacy services may be provided off-site at one or more locations. When the services being performed are related to prescription fulfillment or processing, the pharmacy or pharmacist must comply with the following:

- Long-term care shared pharmacy services in accordance with RCW 18-64-570

- Central fill shared pharmacy services in accordance with the following conditions:

  o The originating pharmacy must have written policies and procedures outlining the off-site pharmacy services to be provided by the central fill pharmacy, or the off-site pharmacist or pharmacy technician, and the responsibilities of each party

  o The parties must share a secure real-time database or utilize other secure technology, including a private, encrypted connection that allows access by the central pharmacy staff to the information necessary to perform off-site pharmacy services

  o A single prescription may be shared by an originating pharmacy and a central fill pharmacy or off-site pharmacist or pharmacy technician. The fulfillment, processing, and delivery of a prescription by one pharmacy for another pursuant to this section will not be construed as the fulfillment of a transferred prescription or as a wholesale distribution.

6 – e

Per WAC 246-945-332, an initial supply of up to thirty days of current prescriptions for legend drug (noncontrolled) medications or a seven-day supply of current prescriptions for controlled substance medications in Schedules III, IV, and V may be provided to patients during a proclaimed emergency. For a prescription that has expired or has no refills, the pharmacist may dispense a one-time emergency refill of the last dispensed quantity or up to a thirty-day supply of a maintenance medication.

7 - d

Per WAC 246-945-430, the following requirements apply to pharmacies storing, dispensing, and delivering drugs to patients without a pharmacist on-site and are in addition to applicable state and federal laws applying to pharmacies:

- The pharmacy is required to have adequate visual surveillance of the full pharmacy and retain a high-quality recording for a minimum of thirty calendar days.

- Access to a pharmacy by individuals must be limited, authorized, and regularly monitored.

- A visual and audio communication system used to counsel and interact with each patient or patient's caregiver must be clear, secure, and HIPAA-compliant.

- The responsible pharmacy manager or designee shall complete and retain, in accordance with WAC 246-945-005, a monthly in-person inspection of the pharmacy.

- A pharmacist must be capable of being on-site at the pharmacy within three hours if an emergency arises.

- The pharmacy must be closed to the public if any component of the surveillance or visual and audio communication system is malfunctioning, and remain closed until system corrections or repairs are completed or a pharmacist is on-site to oversee pharmacy operations.

8 – a, c, d

Per WAC 246-945-435, hospitals are to create their own policies and procedures regarding dispensing medication in the emergency department when pharmacy services are unavailable.

The responsible pharmacy manager of a hospital or free-standing emergency department may develop policies and procedures to provide discharge medications to patients released from hospital emergency departments during hours when community or outpatient hospital pharmacy services are not available. The policies and procedures must:

- Comply with all requirements of RCW 70.41.480

- Ensure all prepackaged medications are affixed with a label that complies with WAC 246-945-018:

  o Drug name

  o Drug strength

  o Expiration date

- o The manufacturer's name and lot number, if not maintained in a separate record

- o The identity of the pharmacist or provider responsible for the prepackaging, if not maintained in a separate record

- Require oral or electronically transmitted chart orders be verified by the practitioner in writing within seventy-two hours

- Require that the medications distributed as discharge medications are stored in compliance with the laws concerning security and access.

9 – e

Per WAC 246-945-345, upon patient request, a prescription may be transferred within the limits of state and federal law. In addition:

- Sufficient information needs to be exchanged in the transfer of a prescription to maintain an auditable trail, as well as all elements of a valid prescription.

- Pharmacies sharing a secure real-time database are not required to transfer prescription information for dispensing.

- Prescriptions must be transferred by electronic means or facsimile except in emergency situations.

10 – e

Previously, using an electronic record-keeping system was optional for a pharmacy. The new rule, WAC 246-945-417, mandates that pharmacies use electronic record-keeping systems.

Record-keeping rules are slightly different for health care entities (HCE) and hospital pharmacy associated clinics (HPAC). HCEs and HPACs may use a paper record-keeping procedure per WAC 246-945-418.

11 – b

Per WAC 246-945-030 and WAC 246-945-031, ephedrine products are classified as legend drugs. Products containing ephedrine or its salts in the amount of 25 mg or less per solid dosage unit or per 5 ml of liquid forms in combination with other ingredients in therapeutic amounts are exempt from legend classification.

12 – e

Per WAC 246-945-173, for an expired pharmacist license, all of these are required if the license is expired for three years or more. On the other hand, if the license is expired for three years or more but the pharmacist has been in practice in another state, then the pharmacist will submit verification of practice in another state and take the Washington state MPJE (the NAPLEX is not required in this case).

13 – e
Per WAC 246-945-025, no person, partnership, corporation, association, or agency shall advertise controlled substances for sale to the general public in any manner that promotes or tends to promote the use or abuse of those drugs. Controlled substances cannot be physically displayed to the public.

14 – e
Per WAC 246-945-031, ephedrine is considered a legend (prescription only) drug if the ephedrine content is over 25mg per solid dosage unit or per 5mL liquid. If the content is 25mg or less, then it is exempt. For example, Primatene contains less than 25mg of ephedrine per tablet, so it can be sold over the counter without a prescription.

15 – d
Washington State law (RCW 69.75.020) states that a person needs to be at least 18 years old in order to purchase any product containing dextromethorphan. The person making the retail sale of a dextromethorphan product must require and obtain proof of age from the purchaser unless the purchaser appears to be at least twenty-five years old. The only exception to the rule is if the purchaser supplies proof that he/she is actively enrolled in the military and presents a valid military ID card.

16 – a
Per WAC 246-945-485, drugs that have been maintained by an institution or facility may be returned and re-dispensed as long as custody is maintained and product integrity is ensured.

A dispensed drug or prescription device must only be accepted for return and reuse as follows:

- Noncontrolled legend drugs that have been maintained in the custody and control of the institutional facility, dispensing pharmacy, or their related facilities under common control may be returned and reused if product integrity can be assured.

- Those that qualify for return under the provisions of chapter 69.70 RCW, which states that prescription drugs or supplies may be accepted and dispensed if the prescription drug is in:

    o Its original sealed and tamper-evident packaging

    o An opened package if it contains single unit doses that remain intact.

17 – a, b, c

All legend drugs are to be dispensed in a child-resistant container as required by federal law unless otherwise authorized. Per WAC 246-945-032, only the prescriber, patient, or patient's representative can authorize dispensing in a container that is not child-resistant. The pharmacist cannot determine or decide for the patient, but can certainly offer.

18 – e

According to WAC 246-945-435 and RCW 70.41.480, policies and procedures are to be implemented by the hospital pharmacy manager. The law limits dispensing to no more than a 48-hour supply of emergency medication. If community or hospital pharmacy services will not be available within that 48-hour period, policy can allow additional dispensing to ensure continuity of care. In no case may the policy allow a supply exceeding 96 hours be dispensed.

19 – d

Per WAC 246-945-162, applicants must complete seven hours of AIDS education for pharmacist licensure. The applicant is exempt from this requirement if they are a graduate of a commission-accredited school or college of pharmacy since the curriculum satisfies this requirement.

20 – b

Per facility standards listed in WAC 246-945-410, facilities need to designate a responsible pharmacy manager. The manager must be designated by the date of opening and within 30 calendar days of a vacancy. The pharmacy manager has the responsibility to assure that the area(s) in the facility where drugs are stored, compounded, delivered, or dispensed are operated in compliance with state and federal laws.

21 – d

Per WAC 246-945-178 and WAC 246-945-990, the pharmacist license renewal schedule is every 2 years, with the license expiring on the pharmacist's birthdate. A minimum of 30 hours of continuing education is required in that two-year period.

22 – c

Previously with WAC 246-858-060, there were requirements for preceptor certification. There are no longer any requirements for a pharmacist to hold a preceptor certification. Any pharmacist can supervise interns gaining experiential hours for licensure or train pharmacy technicians in an approved technician training program.

23 – a, b, c, d, e

The purpose of the prescription monitoring program (PMP) is to detect and prevent prescription drug abuse. Information from the prescription monitoring program may be used by specific people or groups of people for purposes such as research, investigation, assistance in autopsy, and quality improvement. Per WAC 246-470-060, WAC 246-470-080, and 246-470-082, all of the entities listed may receive PMP information.

24 – a, c, e

Per WAC 246-945-330, a pharmacist may renew a prescription for a noncontrolled legend drug one time in a six-month period when an effort has been made to contact the prescriber and they are not available for authorization under the following conditions:

- The amount dispensed is the quantity on the most recent fill or a thirty-day supply, whichever is less

- The refill is requested by the patient or the patient's agent

- The patient has a chronic medical condition

- No changes have been made to the prescription

- The pharmacist communicates the renewal to the prescriber within one business day.

25 – a

Per WAC 246-945-012, a prescription for a Schedule II drug may not be refilled.

26 – c

Per RCW 18.64A.030, pharmacy assistants cannot refill prescriptions (as can pharmacy technicians). Duties that pharmacy assistants can perform include: typing of prescription labels, filing, refiling, bookkeeping, pricing, stocking, delivery, nonprofessional phone inquiries, and documentation of third-party reimbursements.

In addition, per WAC 246-945-315, a pharmacist may delegate the following tasks to pharmacy assistants:

- Prepackage and label drugs for subsequent use in the prescription dispensing operations

- Count, pour, and label for individual prescriptions

The typing of prescription labels is typing by a typewriter, not entering data into the medication record system. Also, be careful not to confuse "filing" with "filling [prescriptions]." Be careful not to confuse "refiling" with "refilling." Pharmacy assistants may file and refile things like documents.

27 – d

Per RCW 8-64-570, where a pharmacy uses shared pharmacy services to have a second pharmacy provide a first dose or partial fill of a prescription or drug order to meet a patient's or resident's immediate needs, the second supplying pharmacy may dispense the first dose or partially filled prescription on a satellite basis without the outsourcing pharmacy being required to fully transfer the prescription to the supplying pharmacy. The supplying pharmacy must retain a copy of the prescription or order on file, a copy of the dispensing record or fill, and must notify the outsourcing pharmacy of the service and quantity provided.

28 – a, b, c, d

Per WAC 246-945-230, if an existing licensed pharmacy is remodeled, the commission must be notified and a facility inspection fee must be paid but a new pharmacy license application does not have to be completed. In addition, the commission licenses a facility that:

- Submits a completed application

- Pays the applicable fees

- Undergoes an inspection by the commission if the facility is located in Washington

- Obtains a controlled substances registration from the commission and is registered with the DEA if the facility intends to possess or distribute controlled substances.

Once an initial license is issued, a licensed facility must:

- Notify the commission and pay a facility inspection fee in lieu of paying an original license fee for modifications or remodels.

- Submit a new application and pay the original license fee if the facility changes location to a different address. If located in Washington, a facility may not relocate prior to the inspection of the new premises.

- Notify the commission and pay the original license fee whenever there is a change in ownership. Change in ownership includes changes in:

  o Business or organizational structure such as a change from sole proprietorship to a corporation

  o Change of more than fifty percent ownership in a corporation.

29 – d

Per WAC 246-945-025, a pharmacy may advertise prescription drugs provided certain conditions are met. The advertising must comply with all state and federal laws. The advertising is solely directed towards providing consumers with drug price information and cannot promote the use of a prescription drug to the public.

A drug price advertisement must contain:

- The proprietary name of the drug product advertised

- The generic name of the drug product advertised

- The strength of the drug product advertised (if the drug product advertised contains more than one active ingredient and a relevant strength can be associated with it without indicating each active ingredient, the generic name and quantity of each active ingredient is not required)

- The price charged for a specified quantity of the drug product.

30 – d
Per WAC 246-945-011 and RCW 69.50.308, Schedule V controlled substances expire after 6 months from date of issue or after 5 refills, whichever comes first.

31 – c
Per WAC 246-945-011, a pharmacist must verify the validity of a prescription prior to dispensing. A prescription is considered invalid for the following reasons:

- The prescription shows evidence of alteration, erasure, or addition by any person other than the person who wrote it

- The prescription does not contain the minimum required information (WAC 246-945-010)

- The prescription is expired

  o The prescription is for a controlled substance listed in Schedule II through V and the date of dispensing is *more than six months* after the prescription's date of issue.

  o The prescription is for a noncontrolled legend drug or OTC drug and the date of dispensing is more than twelve months after the prescription's date of issue.

- The prescription for a controlled substance does not comply with requirements in the Uniform Controlled Substance Act (RCW 69.50.308)

Depending on the prescription, certain information may be added or changed to make the prescription valid. For example, the directions for use may be added to a controlled substance prescription after discussion with the prescriber.

32 – a

Per WAC 246-945-455, emergency kit drugs shall be accessible only to licensed healthcare professionals.

33 – b

Per WAC 246-945-345:

- Upon patient request, a prescription may be transferred within the limits of state and federal law

- Sufficient information needs to be exchanged in the transfer of a prescription to maintain an auditable trail, as well as all elements of a valid prescription

- Pharmacies sharing a secure real-time database are not required to transfer prescription information for dispensing

- Prescriptions must be transferred by electronic means or facsimile, except in emergency situations.

34 – a

Per WAC 246-945-035, the possession, distribution, or dispensing of drug samples is prohibited in retail pharmacies and wholesale distributors. However, a pharmacy in a hospital or health care entity that receives drug samples at the request of an authorized practitioner may distribute drug samples.

A health care entity is defined as any organization or business entity that provides diagnostic, medical, surgical, or dental treatment and/or rehabilitative care.

35 – a, c

Per WAC 246-945-017, minimum requirements for hospital inpatient labels include:

- Drug name (generic and/or trade) and strength, when applicable

- A compounded product must meet the applicable labeling requirements of USP chapters <795>, <797>, <800>, and <825>.

36 – c

Per WAC 246-945-011, prescriptions for non-controlled legend drugs or over-the-counter medications expire after 12 months from date of issue.

37 – b

Per WAC 246-945-020, the record retention period for prescription and refill records is at least 2 years.

38 – c

Per WAC 246-945-420, pharmacies operating without a pharmacist are required to maintain a perpetual inventory record. Records for Schedule II controlled substances must be maintained separately from all other records. Controlled substance records must be kept for two years.

Controlled substance records may include invoices, receipts, orders, distribution records, emergency transfer records, and DEA form 106; all must be kept for two years. Per WAC 246-945-420, controlled substance inventory is conducted every two years.

39 – a, b, d

Per RCW 18.64.265, a partial fill of a Schedule II controlled substance is permitted if the partial fill is requested by the patient or prescriber and the total quantity requested in all partial fillings does not exceed the quantity prescribed. A pharmacist cannot decide for the patient to partial fill the prescription, but could discuss it for the patient to decide.

In addition, WAC 246-945-013 applies partial fills to non-controlled legend drugs and Schedule III–V controlled substances.

40 – b

The prescriber's name is required. Per WAC 246-945-010, the minimum elements required on a prescription for a non-controlled legend drug are:

- Prescriber's name

- Name of patient, authorized entity, or animal name and species

- Date of issuance

- Drug name, strength, and quantity

- Directions for use

- Number of refills, if any

- Instruction on whether or not a therapeutically equivalent generic drug or interchangeable biological product may be substituted, unless substitution is permitted under a prior-consent authorization

- Prescriber's manual or electronic signature (can be an authorized agent)

If the prescription is written, it must be written on a tamper-resistant prescription pad or paper approved by the commission.

41 – c

Per WAC 246-945-011, prescriptions for Schedule II controlled substances are valid for 6 months from date of issue. After 6 months, the prescription is considered expired.

42 – e

Per WAC 246-945-010, a prescription for a controlled substance must include all the information required on a non-controlled prescription, plus:

- Patient's address

- Dosage form

- Prescriber's address

- Prescriber's DEA registration number

- Any other requirements listed in 21 C.F.R., Chapter II

43 – b, c, d

Per WAC 246-945-045 and RCW 69.50.402, in addition to any FDA-approved indication, Schedule II stimulants may only be prescribed for certain disease treatments or as part of approved clinical investigation.

Indications for which Schedule II stimulants may be prescribed include:

- Moderate to severe binge eating disorder in adults

- Narcolepsy

- Hyperkinesis

- Drug-induced brain dysfunction

- Epilepsy

- Differential diagnostic psychiatric evaluation of depression

- Depression shown to be refractory to other therapeutic modalities

- Multiple sclerosis

44 – a, b, c, d, e

Per WAC 246-945-018, all of these are required on the label of prepackaged medications. Prepackaged medications also include medications dispensed in a unit dose form and medications dispensed by a pharmacy to a long-term care facility.

45 – a

Per WAC 246-945-016 and RCW 69.41.050, the prescriber's address is not required on the prescription label.

WAC 246-945-016 requires the minimum requirements as listed in RCW 69.41.050:

- Name and address of the dispensing pharmacy

- Prescription number

- Name of the prescriber

- Prescriber's directions

- Name and strength of the medication

- Name of the patient

- Date of dispensing

- Expiration date

As well as these additional requirements:

- Drug quantity

- The number of refills remaining, if any

- The statement "Warning: State or federal law prohibits transfer of this drug to any person other than the person for whom it was prescribed" (except when dispensing to an animal, when a warning sufficient to convey "for veterinary use only" may be used)

- The name and species of the patient, if a veterinary prescription

- The name of the facility or entity authorized by law to possess a legend drug, if the patient is the facility or entity.

46 – a

Per RCW 69.41.042 and WAC 246-945-020, invoice records need to be kept for two years.

47 – d

A pharmacy technician may enter prescriptions into the computer. Technicians are also allowed to fill prescriptions, compound medications, and call a prescriber's office for refill authorization.

Per WAC 246-945-320, there are several pharmacist responsibilities that cannot be delegated to pharmacy ancillary personnel (technicians and assistants), including receiving and transferring verbal prescriptions from a physician's office (an exception is refill authorization), consultation with the patient regarding the prescription, interpreting data from the patient medication record system, consulting a prescriber, final verification of dispensed drugs, patient counseling, drug or biologic substitutions, and refusal to dispense drugs or devices based on restricted distribution regulations.

48 – d

A poison register is a register kept by a pharmacist that records the names of people to whom poison has been made available. Per RCW 69.38.030, a purchaser must disclose the purpose for which the poison is being purchased. The poison register will maintain the following information:

- The date and hour of the sale

- The full name and home address of the purchaser

- The kind and quantity of poison sold

- The purpose for which the poison is being purchased

The purchaser must present to the seller identification which contains the purchaser's photograph and signature. No sale may be made unless the seller is satisfied that the purchaser's representations are true and that the poison will be used for a lawful purpose. Both the purchaser and the seller must sign the poison register entry.

49 – e

Per WAC 246-945-460, there is no longer a maximum pharmacist to technician ratio of 1:3. The pharmacy manager is to use their professional judgement to determine appropriate staffing levels for the practice setting.

This means a pharmacist can potentially oversee the work of more than 3 technicians, if appropriate.

50 – b

Per RCW 69.51A.260, the maximum number of marijuana plants grown or located in any one housing unit is 15 plants. This applies even if multiple qualifying patients or designated providers reside in the same housing unit.

51 – b, d

The commission considers the function of transferring a noncontrolled prescription by electronic means (including facsimile) to be a nondiscretionary function associated with the practice of pharmacy that is delegable to a pharmacy technician pursuant to WAC 246-945-315.

However, the transfer of verbal prescriptions to another pharmacy cannot be delegated to a pharmacy technician. Pharmacy technicians are NOT permitted at any time to transfer verbal or non-verbal controlled substance prescriptions according to the DEA and the commission's promulgated rules.

52 – e

According to WAC Chapter 246-978, all of the statements are correct. The attending physician may not be one of the witnesses. "Competent" means that the patient has the ability to make and communicate an informed decision to health care providers. The attending physician ensures that the patient is making an informed decision by providing information on the patient's medical diagnosis, prognosis, potential risks of taking the medication to end his or her life, and the probable result of taking the medication to be prescribed.

53 – e

Per WAC 246-945-090, a Medicare-approved dialysis center may dispense sterile heparin, sterile potassium chloride, dialysate, and sterile sodium chloride, in cases or full shelf package lots, to their home dialysis patients if prescribed by a physician. Epoetin alfa, which treats anemia, is not included within this law.

54 – e

Per RCW 70.225.020, all of the statements accurately describe the purpose of the prescription monitoring program.

55 – a, b, c, d, e

Per RCW 70.225.020, all of the answers, plus the date of dispensing, are required to be submitted to the prescription monitoring program (PMP).

56 – e

Per WAC 246-945-205, applicants for pharmacy technician certification need to be at least 18 years old and hold a high school diploma or GED. Applicants need to complete 8 hours of guided study of Washington state and federal pharmacy law and provide proof of completion of a pharmacy technician training program.

Acceptable documentation of completing a commission-approved pharmacy technician program includes:

- Signed documentation from an on-the-job training program

- Transcripts or a diploma for formal academic or college programs

- Documentation if training was provided by a branch of the federal armed forces

Applicants must pass a national certification examination approved by the commission within one year of completing the training program and applying for certification.

57 – a, b, c, d, e
Per WAC 246-945-170, all of the statements are correct. A pharmacist with a temporary license has full scope to practice pharmacy but does not qualify to be a responsible pharmacist manager.

58 – c
Per RCW 18.64.140, a copy of the pharmacist's current license must be displayed openly in any licensed pharmacy location where the pharmacist is practicing. This would mean that pharmacists who work in several locations should have a copy for each location. There are currently no laws that explicitly prohibit obscuring the pharmacist's address for privacy. Washington's Public Records Act could protect a licensee from having to disclose address information to the public.

59 – a
Per WAC 246-945-178, a one-time training in suicide screening and referral is required in the first pharmacist license renewal cycle after January 1, 2017. The training must be at least 3 hours long. It must be selected from the Department of Health's list of approved suicide prevention training programs and the core content must include information on:

- Screening and referral

- Assessment of issues related to imminent harm via lethal means.

60 – a, b, c, d
Per RCW 70.225.020, the department shall establish and maintain a prescription monitoring program (PMP) to monitor the prescribing and dispensing of all Schedule II, III, IV, and V controlled substances and any additional drugs identified by the Pharmacy Quality Assurance Commission as demonstrating a potential for abuse. Only drugs dispensed for more than a one-day supply are reported.

Pseudoephedrine is tracked using NPLEx, not the PMP.

61 – c

Per WAC 246-945-040, in the event of a significant loss or theft, two copies of DEA 106 (report of theft or loss of controlled substances) must be transmitted to the federal authorities and a copy must be sent to the commission.

62 – e

Per RCW 69.51A.050, the lawful possession of medical marijuana cannot result in forfeiture or seizure of the qualifying patient's property. The state is also not responsible for any deleterious outcomes from the use of medical marijuana.

Additionally, per RCW 69.51A.040, a qualifying patient or designated provider needs to be entered into the medical marijuana authorization database and needs to hold a valid recognition card. The qualifying patient or designated provider will present the recognition card to law enforcement officers when applicable.

A copy of the recognition card and qualifying patient or designated provider's contact information needs to be posted prominently next to any medical marijuana plants and products in the residence.

63 – b

Per WAC 246-945-020, records must be maintained for at least 2 years.

64 – a, c

Normally fax orders for Schedule II controlled substances are not permissible, except if the patient is in a long-term care facility or hospice program. Per RCW 69.50.308, a pharmacy may dispense Schedule II narcotic substances pursuant to a facsimile (fax) order under the following circumstances:

- The facsimile prescription is transmitted by a practitioner to the pharmacy

- The facsimile prescription is for a patient in a hospice or long-term care facility

- The practitioner or agent notes on the facsimile prescription that the patient is a long-term care or hospice patient.

65 – c

The Washington Board of Pharmacy consists of 15 members: 10 pharmacists, 1 pharmacy technician, and 4 public members. Pharmacist members must be actively practicing.

66 – d

Per WAC 246-945-178, A pharmacist must complete the equivalent of 3.0 of CPE hours (equal to thirty contact hours) administered by an ACPE-accredited provider every two-year license renewal cycle.

67 – c

Per WAC 246-470-030, a dispenser must submit data when dispensing a controlled substance. This includes the name of person picking up or dropping off the prescription, as verified by valid photographic identification when practicable.

68 – d

Out-of-state prescriptions from optometrists cannot be filled. Out-of-state prescriptions are allowed from only the following prescribers: physicians (MD or DO), podiatric physicians (DPM), dentists (DDS, DMD), veterinarians (DVM), advanced registered nurse practitioners (ARNP), and physician assistants (PA).

69 – b, c, d

WAC 246-945-005 covers self-inspections:

- The responsible pharmacy manager, or equivalent manager, is required to conduct an annual self-inspection of the pharmaceutical firm

  o Self-inspection worksheets are provided by the commission

  o The self-inspection must be completed within the month of March each year

- The responsible pharmacy manager must sign and date the completed self-inspection worksheet(s)

  o Worksheets must be maintained for two years from the date of completion

- When a change in responsible pharmacy manager occurs, the new responsible pharmacy manager must conduct a self-inspection

  o The self-inspection must be completed within thirty days of becoming responsible pharmacy manager

  o The completed worksheets must be maintained for two years from the date of completion.

70 – b

The signature may be kept as a hardcopy with the transaction number recorded in a logbook. Additionally, if the tracking system is temporarily unavailable, the retailer may record all the information needed and enter it into the monitoring system within 72 hours of the system becoming operational. Per WAC 246-945-078, a retailer must enter and electronically transmit the following information to the methamphetamine precursor tracking system prior to completion of the transaction:

- Date and time of the intended purchase

- Product description

- Quantity of product to be sold including:

    o Total grams of restricted product per box

    o Number of boxes per transaction

- Purchaser's information including:

    o Full name as it appears on the acceptable identification

    o Date of birth

    o The address as it appears on the photo identification or the current address if the form of photo identification used does not contain the purchaser's address. The address information must include the house number, street, city, state, and zip code

    o Form of photo identification presented by the purchaser, including the issuing agency of the acceptable identification, and the identification number appearing on the identification

    o Purchaser's signature

        ▪ If the retailer is not able to secure an electronic signature, the retailer shall maintain a hard copy of a signature logbook consisting of each purchaser's signature and the transaction number provided by the methamphetamine precursor tracking system

- The full name or initials of the individual conducting the transaction

- Other information as required by the methamphetamine precursor tracking system database

If a transaction occurs during a time when the methamphetamine precursor tracking system is temporarily unavailable due to power outage or other technical difficulties, the retailer shall record the information required in this section in a written logbook for entry into the methamphetamine precursor tracking system within seventy-two hours of the system becoming operational.

71 – b

Per WAC 246-945-325 the pharmacist must offer to counsel all patients:

- Upon the initial fill of a prescription for a new or change of therapy.

- When the pharmacist using their professional judgment determines counseling is necessary to promote safe and effective use and to facilitate an appropriate therapeutic outcome for that patient.

Per WAC 246-945-325 patient counseling is a nondelegable task performed by a pharmacist.

72 – b, c, d

All legend drugs shall be dispensed in a child-resistant container as required by federal law or regulation unless:

- Authorization is received from the prescriber to dispense in a container that is not child-resistant

- Authorization is obtained from the patient or a representative of the patient to dispense in a container that is not child-resistant

No pharmacist or pharmacy employee may designate themselves as the patient's agent.

However, there are exceptions, such as with sublingual nitroglycerin, sublingual and chewable forms of isosorbide dinitrate 10mg or less, conjugated estrogen tablets (birth control) containing not more than 32.0 mg of drug, and more.

Refer to Poison Prevention Packaging 16 C.F.R., Part 1700 for the full, detailed list.

73 – e

The pharmacy owner must notify the Pharmacy Commission at least 30 days prior to the anticipated closing date. The owner must provide a written statement containing:

- The date the pharmacy will close

- The names and addresses of the persons who will have custody of prescription files, bulk compounding records, repackaging records, and the controlled substance inventory

- The names and addresses of any persons who will acquire the legend drugs, if known

More information needs to be provided to the commission after the pharmacy has closed, which is stated in WAC 246-945-480.

74 – a, b, d
Per WAC 246-945-335, upon patient consent, a pharmacist may adapt drugs as specified in this rule, provided that the prescriber has not indicated that adaptation is not permitted.

- Change quantity. A pharmacist may change the quantity of medication prescribed if:

  o The prescribed quantity or package size is not commercially available

  o The change in quantity is related to a change in dosage form

  o The change is intended to dispense up to the total amount authorized by the prescriber, including refills in accordance

  o The change extends a maintenance drug for the limited quantity necessary to coordinate a patient's refills in a medication synchronization program

- Change dosage form. A pharmacist may change the dosage form of the prescription if it is in the best interest of patient care, so long as the prescriber's directions are also modified to equate to an equivalent amount of drug dispensed as prescribed.

- Complete missing information. A pharmacist may complete missing information on a prescription if there is evidence to support the change.

A pharmacist who adapts a prescription in accordance with these rules must document the adaptation in the patient's record.

75 – c, d, e
Per WAC 246-945-340, A pharmacist may substitute a drug product or a biologic product when any of the following applies:

- The substitution is permitted by RCW 69.41.120 (the prescription did not indicate "DISPENSE AS WRITTEN")

- The substitution is permitted by a formulary developed by an interdisciplinary team of an institutional facility

  o An employee or contractor of the institutional facility prescribed the drug or biologic product to be substituted

- o The interdisciplinary team was composed of a nonpharmacist prescriber listed in RCW 69.41.030 and a pharmacist

- o The formulary is readily retrievable by the pharmacist

- The substitution is otherwise permitted by law.

76 – a, b, d, e

Per WAC 246-470-037, a facility that is subject to the prescription monitoring program integration mandate requirement and is experiencing an economic hardship, technological limitation, or another exceptional circumstance may submit an attestation to the department for a waiver from the integration mandate.

- The attestation must be submitted on forms provided by the department. The waiver is deemed granted upon submission

- The facility is exempt from the prescription monitoring program integration mandate for the calendar year

  - o For economic hardship and technical limitation, a facility may submit up to three annual attestations

  - o There is no limit on the number of other exceptional circumstance waivers that a facility may submit

- A facility may submit an attestation for a waiver from the mandate due to:

  - o Economic hardship in the following circumstances:

    - ▪ A bankruptcy in the previous year

    - ▪ Opening a new practice after January 1, 2020

    - ▪ Operating a low-income clinic, that is defined as a clinic serving a minimum of thirty percent Medicaid patients

    - ▪ Intent to discontinue operating in Washington prior to December 31, 2022

- Technological limitations outside the control of the facility group in the following circumstance:

- Integration of an electronic health records system with the PMP through a method approved by the department is in process but has not yet been completed

- Other exceptional circumstances include:

  - Providing services as a free clinic

  - The internet speed or bandwidth required to integrate an electronic health record with the prescription monitoring program through a method approved by the department is not available

  - The technology to connect the electronic health record of the entity requesting the waiver to the prescription monitoring program through a method approved by the department does not exist

  - Fewer than one hundred prescriptions for Schedule II–V drugs are generated in a calendar year

  - Unforeseen circumstances that stress the practitioner or health care system in such a way that compliance is not possible. Examples may include, but are not limited to, natural disasters, widespread health care emergencies, unforeseen barriers to integration, or unforeseen events that result in a statewide emergency.

77 – a

Per WAC 246-945-051, synthetic cannabinoids, also known as Spice and K2, are Schedule I controlled substances in Washington state. Substituted cathinones (bath salts) are also listed under Schedule I.

78 – b

Per WAC 246-945-480, when a pharmacy is closing, the pharmacy must report to the Pharmacy Quality Assurance Commission no later than 30 days prior to closing. The pharmacy needs to provide the following information:

- The date the pharmacy will close

- The names and addresses of persons who will have custody of prescription files, records, invoices, and controlled substance inventory records

- The names and addresses of any person(s) who will acquire any legend drugs from the pharmacy, if known at the time.

79 – c

Per WAC 246-945-220, 2.0 continuing pharmacy education (CPE) hours, which equals 20 contact hours, are required every two-year license renewal cycle.

80 – c

Per RCW 69.43.110, the maximum amount of pseudoephedrine that can be sold over the counter to an individual in one day is 3.6 grams. The rule applies to over-the-counter sale and not prescription sale.

81 – e

Per RCW 69.43.110, a pharmacy may not sell more than 9 grams of over-the-counter pseudoephedrine products to an individual within a 30-day period.

82 – a

Per WAC 246-945-087, if pseudoephedrine is dispensed pursuant to a prescription (rather than an over-the-counter sale), then it does not need to be reported to NPLEx.

83 – c

DEA Form 222 is used for the distribution, purchase, or transfer of a Schedule II controlled substance. It is important to note that Form 222 is used for Schedule II substances and not Schedule III–V.

84 – d

Per WAC 246-945-077, the purchaser must be at least 18 years old, not 21 years old. Acceptable forms of identification are as follows: a valid driver's license or permit; a United States Armed Forces identification card; a merchant marine identification card; an identification card issued by any foreign, federal or state government; an official passport; or an enrollment card issued by a federally recognized Indian tribe.

Additionally, per WAC 246-945-078, each retailer must enter and electronically transmit the following information to the methamphetamine precursor tracking system prior to completion of the transaction:

- Sale transaction information including:

  - Date and time of the intended purchase

  - Product description

  - Quantity of product to be sold including:

    - Total grams of restricted product per box

- Number of boxes per transaction

- Purchaser's information including:

  ○ Full name as it appears on the acceptable identification

  ○ Date of birth

  ○ The address as it appears on the photo identification or the current address if the form of photo identification used does not contain the purchaser's address. The address information must include the house number, street, city, state, and zip code

  ○ Form of photo identification presented by the purchaser, including the issuing agency of the acceptable identification, and the identification number appearing on the identification

- Purchaser's signature. If the retailer is not able to secure an electronic signature, the retailer shall maintain a hard copy of a signature logbook consisting of each purchaser's signature and the transaction number provided by the methamphetamine precursor tracking system.

- The full name or initials of the individual conducting the transaction

- Other information as required by the methamphetamine precursor tracking system database.

85 – c

In Washington, an individual may purchase syringes/needles without a prescription. The sale of syringes/needles is not restricted to the pharmacy in Washington (in a few states, the sale of syringes/needles is restricted to the pharmacy).

Per Chapter 70.115 RCW, for the retail sale of syringes and needles, the retailer shall satisfy themselves that the device will be used for the legal use intended. The retailer is not required to sell syringes and needles to any person.

In other words, the retailer may refuse to sell syringes/needles depending on the circumstances.

86 – a, b, c

Per WAC 246-903-030, in order for a pharmacist to qualify as a nuclear pharmacist, he or she must meet the minimum standards of training. In addition, they must be licensed in Washington state.

They must submit their certification of training to the board, which can include either:

- Certification of 6 months of on-the-job training

- Completion of a nuclear pharmacy training program from an accredited college of pharmacy

- Completion of a nuclear pharmacy training program from an unaccredited college of pharmacy, but with approval of the board.

87 – d
Per 21 U.S.C. Sec. 829, in an emergency situation where a Schedule II controlled substance is partially dispensed, the remaining fill shall be dispensed no later than 72 hours after the prescription is issued.

88 – a, b, c, d, e
All of these entities are required to be licensed as a wholesaler in Washington State. The wholesaler license applies to every wholesaler who engages in wholesale distribution into, out of, or within Washington state.

Per WAC 246-945-246, the full list of entities that are required to be licensed as a wholesaler are:

- In-state and out-of-state pharmaceutical wholesalers

- Out-of-state manufacturers that distribute or sell drugs into Washington

- Virtual wholesalers

- Out-of-state virtual manufacturers that distribute or sell drugs into Washington

- Outsourcing facilities required to be registered with the FDA as an outsourcing facility which are located in Washington, or which distribute or sell drugs into Washington

- Reverse distributors.

89 – c
Per WAC 246-945-330, pharmacists are permitted to renew a prescription for a non-controlled legend drug once in a six-month period if the prescriber is unable to be reached. The refill quantity must equal the most recent quantity dispensed or a 30-day supply, whichever is less. The pharmacist must also notify the prescriber of the prescription refill within 1 business day.

90 – d

A pharmacist may substitute a drug product or a biologic product when the substitution is permitted by a formulary of an institutional facility. The following criteria must be met:

- An employee or contractor of the institutional facility prescribed the drug or biologic product to be substituted

- The interdisciplinary team was composed of a non-pharmacist prescriber and a pharmacist

- The formulary is readily retrievable by the pharmacist.

91 – d

WAC 246-945-415 permits after-hours delivery and returns. Filled prescriptions may be picked up or returned for delivery by authorized personnel when the pharmacy is closed for business if the prescriptions are placed in a secured delivery area outside of the drug storage area.

The secured area must be part of the licensed pharmacy. The secured area must also be equipped with adequate security, including an alarm or comparable monitoring system. Access to the secured delivery area needs to be addressed in the policies and procedures of the pharmacy (the pharmacy manager is responsible for developing these policies and procedures).

92 – b

Physicians do not have restrictions on prescribing authority. Naturopathic doctors can only prescribe certain controlled substances. Optometrists cannot prescribe oral steroids or Schedule II controlled substances except for hydrocodone combination products. Veterinarians can only prescribe for animal treatment. Certified nurse anesthetists can only prescribe legend and Schedule II–IV substances for anesthesia per protocol.

93 – d

Per WAC 246-470-030, a dispenser must provide to the department the dispensing information for all scheduled II, III, IV, and V controlled substances and for drugs identified by the pharmacy quality assurance commission. Only drugs dispensed for more than one day use must be reported. Prescription drug monitoring program data submission requirements do not apply to:

- Correctional institutions or pharmacies operated for the purpose of providing medications to offenders in the state ("prison pharmacies").

- Medications provided to patients receiving inpatient services (at the hospital), including the hospital's surgery areas.

94 – a, b, d, e

Per WAC 246-945-455, in order for drugs to be stored in a designated area outside the pharmacy, including in floor stock, in an emergency cabinet, in an emergency kit, or as emergency outpatient drug delivery from an emergency department at a registered institutional facility, the following conditions must be met:

- Drugs stored in such a manner shall remain under the control of, and be routinely monitored by, the supplying pharmacy

- The supplying pharmacy shall develop and implement policies and procedures to: prevent and detect unauthorized access; document drugs used, returned and wasted; and complete regular inventory procedures

- Access must be limited to health care professionals licensed under the chapters specified in RCW 18.130.040 acting within their scope, and nursing students as provided in WAC 246-945-450

- The area must be equipped with security to protect from diversion or tampering

- The facility must be able to possess and store drugs

This does not include the use of an emergency kit or supplemental dose kit by nursing homes and hospice programs, as they must comply with RCW 18.64.560.

95 – c

Per WAC 246-945-010, if a practitioner authorizes an emergency oral prescription for a Schedule II controlled substance, the practitioner must deliver a signed prescription to the pharmacy within 7 days. If the prescription is delivered by mail, it must be postmarked within the 7-day period. The pharmacist must make a note on the prescription that it was filled on an emergency basis.

96 – e

Per WAC 246-945-335, with patient consent, a pharmacist may:

- Change quantity. They may change the quantity of medication prescribed if:

  o The prescribed quantity or package size is not commercially available

  o The change in quantity is related to a change in dosage form

  o The change is intended to dispense up to the total amount authorized by the prescriber, including refills in accordance with RCW 18.64.520 (i.e., changing to a 90-day supply) o   The change extends a maintenance drug for the limited quantity necessary to coordinate a patient's refills in a medication synchronization program in accordance with RCW 48.43.096

- Change dosage form. The form may be changed if it is in the best interest of patient care, so long as the prescriber's directions are also modified to equate to an equivalent amount of drug dispensed as prescribed

- Complete missing information. A pharmacist may complete missing information on a prescription if there is evidence to support the change

A pharmacist who adapts a prescription in accordance with these rules must document the adaptation in the patient's record.

97 – a
Per WAC 246-470-030, controlled substance dispensing dates shall be submitted to the program electronically not later than one business day from the date of dispensing. If the dispenser has not dispensed any drugs that require PMP reporting, then within 7 days the dispenser needs to report that no drugs requiring reporting were dispensed.

98 – a, b, c, d, e
Per RCW 70.54.440, an authorized entity includes any entity or organization in which allergens are capable of causing anaphylaxis. Authorized entities include, but are not limited to: restaurants, recreation camps, youth sports leagues, amusement parks, colleges, universities, and sports arenas.

99 – e
A pharmacist may not prescribe buprenorphine for opioid dependency treatment. Previously, only MDs and DOs were permitted to prescribe buprenorphine for opioid dependency treatment. Now, NPs and PAs may also prescribe buprenorphine for opioid dependency treatment if they have completed training and applied for a waiver.

100 – a, b, d
Prescriptions written by out-of-state MDs, DOs, DDSs, DPMs, DMDs, DVMs, ARNPs and "physician assistants" may be dispensed. Dispensing is not permitted for other out-of-state prescribers.

Prescriptions written by MDs, DOs, DDSs, DPMs, DMDs, DVMs, ARNPs and "physician assistants" from British Columbia may be dispensed, except for controlled substances, since they are not DEA registrants.

Contact Us

Pharmacy Testing Solutions is committed to publishing high-quality, accurate test prep materials. We have had multiple pharmacists review this material as well as a copyeditor. However, despite our best efforts, we realize that an occasional error may occur. If you encounter anything that appears to be incorrect, please contact us!

We will immediately review the issue and publish a correction if necessary. This will help to ensure that our content is 100% accurate for future students. And we will also send you a nice reward for any significant errors that are brought to our attention. You may contact us at: PharmacyTestingSolutions@gmail.com.

Thanks for choosing our MPJE review book!

Made in United States
Troutdale, OR
05/19/2024

19975539R00064